Looking
North for
Health

EDITED BY
**Arnold Bennett
and Orvill Adams**

**Families USA Foundation
Ron Pollack, executive director**

FOREWORD BY
Senator John D. Rockefeller IV

Looking North for Health

WHAT WE CAN LEARN FROM CANADA'S HEALTH CARE SYSTEM

 Jossey-Bass Publishers
San Francisco

Substantial discounts on bulk quantities of Jossey-Bass books are available to corporations, professional associations, and other organizations. For details and discount information, contact the special sales department at Jossey-Bass Inc., Publishers. (415) 433-1740; Fax (415) 433-0499.

For sales outside the United States, contact Maxwell Macmillan International Publishing Group, 866 Third Avenue, New York, New York 10022.

Manufactured in the United States of America

The paper used in this book is acid-free and meets the State of California requirements for recycled paper (50 percent recycled waste, including 10 percent postconsumer waste), which are the strictest guidelines for recycled paper currently in use in the United States.

10% POST CONSUMER WASTE

The ink in this book is either soy- or vegetable-based and during the printing process emits fewer than half the volatile organic compounds (VOCs) emitted by petroleum-based ink.

Chapter One is an edited version of Evans, R. G. "We'll Take Care of It for You: Health Care in the Canadian Community." *Daedalus: Journal of the American Academy of Arts and Sciences,* Fall 1988, *117*(4), 155–189. Reprinted with permission.

The quoted material in Chapter Three is used with permission of Allan S. Detsky, W. Vickery Stoughton, and William Fisher.

Library of Congress Cataloging-in-Publication Data

Looking north for health : what we can learn from Canada's health care system / edited by Arnold Bennett, Orvill Adams ; foreword by John D. Rockefeller IV. — 1st ed.
    p.   cm. — (The Jossey-Bass health series)
    Includes bibliographic references and index.
    ISBN 1-55542-516-X
    1. National health insurance—Canada. 2. Medical care—Canada.
I. Bennett, Arnold. II. Adams, Orvill. III. Families USA Foundation. IV. Series.
RA412.5.C3L56 1993
362.1'0971—dc20   92-41382
                                           CIP

FIRST EDITION
HB Printing   10 9 8 7 6 5 4 3 2 1   *Code 9326*

The Jossey-Bass Health Series

Contents

Foreword

It wasn't easy for Jim and Rebecca Schienle to decide to put Jim's mother in a nursing home. The increasingly debilitating effects of Alzheimer's disease had brought her to live with them a year earlier. The whole family made sacrifices to care for her at home. The teenage boys moved to the den to give their ailing grandmother a room of her own. Rebecca quit her job to care for her mother-in-law. The reduced family income, coupled with expenses for the older woman's care, nearly cost the Schienles their home.

Ultimately, the Schienles saw no option other than institutionalization for Jim's mother. Like all adult children making such decisions, they are plagued by doubt and guilt. Mr. Schienle agonizes over whether he could have done more to reciprocate for the care his mother gave him while he was growing up.

The Schienles are victims of the lack of home care and adult day-care options available in our current system, services that would provide additional—and humane—choices for families facing a long term care crisis.

I met the Schienles when they described their ordeal to the U.S. Bipartisan Commission on Comprehensive Health Care. This commission, created by Congress to make policy recommendations on comprehensive health and long term care became known as the Pepper Commission when its first chair, the widely revered Senator Claude Pepper of Florida, died during deliberations.

I had the honor of succeeding Senator Pepper as chair. Other members were the late Senator John Heinz (R-Pa.), Senators David Pryor (D-Ark.), David Durenberger (R-Minn.), Edward Kennedy (D-Mass.), and Max Baucus (D-Mont.), Representatives Henry Waxman (D-Calif.), Mary Rose Oakar (D-Ohio), Louis Stokes (D-Ohio), Thomas Tauke (R-Iowa), Pete Stark (D-Calif.), and Willis Gradison (R-Ohio), as well as past president of the American Medical Association James Davis, economist James Balog, and academician John Cogan.

The real tragedy of the Schienles is that they are not unique. As the Commission discovered, millions of families face health and long term care crises. They face painful decisions and make personal sacrifices to care for loved ones. There is virtually no public or private insurance for custodial care at home or in a nursing home in this country. Public support is primarily through the Medicaid program, which was created to provide health care to the very poor; it is available only after people have exhausted their own resources.

Financing problems permeate both the long term care system and the acute care system, stirring fear and anxiety among the tens of millions already excluded from it and the increasing numbers at risk of exclusion:

> Uninsured pregnant women, without access to prenatal care
>
> Workers with preexisting medical conditions that may cost them their health insurance if they change jobs
>
> Workers in small businesses, who can put insurance premiums out of reach for the entire firm with a costly illness
>
> Workers with good coverage, who see their benefits threatened each time they go to the bargaining table

Learning from Other Societies

Part of our distinctly American genius is to learn from other societies and then adapt and improve upon that knowledge in a singularly American style. Our diverse society opens Americans to the rich lessons of other civilizations upon which we, in turn, build and improve. This is truer for our nation, I'm convinced, than for more homogeneous countries.

It makes tremendous sense that we should be interested in the health care experiences of other countries so we can evaluate strengths and weaknesses of various models. Our neighbor to the north offers a valuable opportunity to learn from the experiences of a country with which we have notable similarities. We share with Canada basic values and strong traditions of democracy and equality. It is valuable to see how Canada has coped with the same problems of health and long term care that now confront the United States.

With this in mind, I worked with Families USA Foundation, a respected consumer group on issues of health and long term care, to convene Looking North for Health, a forum on Canada's health and long term care systems that was the seed for this book. Families USA invited distinguished health experts from Canada to Washington to share their expertise and experiences with us. Many of them contributed chapters to this excellent book, including one of the creators of the Canadian system, the distinguished former premier of Saskatchewan, Allan E. Blakeney. Also among them are members of the ruling Conservative Party, who have a deep respect for the idea of using government to actively help citizens solve such family problems as the need for affordable health care.

The final chapter, by Families USA's executive director, Ron Pollack, pulls the book together by exploring the lessons we can draw from the Canadian experience.

As researchers thoroughly examine every previous bit of work on a selected topic, we should examine other nations' systems to guide our own transformation. It makes good sense to look at how Canada is coping with its health care system, at what is working and what is not. By understanding the successes and failures of others, we can shape a uniquely American set of comprehensive reforms to control cost, strengthen quality, and assure peace of mind to all of our families.

This book makes an important contribution to this process by giving a truly panoramic view of Canadian health and long term care. It is written in a style that makes it accessible to all Americans who care about the future of our health care system, but with the serious attention to detail that makes it valuable to the expert or scholar, as well.

Roads to Reform

The Pepper Commission developed strong and sensible proposals for health and long term care reform that would guarantee all Americans coverage within a system that both ensures quality and keeps costs down. The Commission recommended development of public policies for acute care and long term care to guarantee Americans of all ages affordable, high-quality care.

The American way of financing health and long term care for our families needs to change. Most Americans agree about that. This book, *Looking North for Health,* is a valuable resource for all who are committed to the reform of America's health and long term care systems. It is especially valuable because it deals with the *entire* continuum of care in Canada, including the Canadians' extraordinary provincial long term care programs, as well as the acute care system.

We must take what we learn from other nations, avoid their errors, match their successes, and make the necessary improvements in our health system to work toward this reasonable goal: ensuring the health care of all Americans while ending the anxieties about cost that now haunt American families.

I look forward to the day when *Canadians* will be able to look *south* for health after we have put together a health care system that is, once again, a source of pride — not anxiety — to Americans.

December 1992   John D. Rockefeller IV
                                             senator from West Virginia

Preface

After the death of Patricia S., *ABC World News Tonight* told her story: Patricia might still be alive if her insurance company had approved the cancer operation her doctor prescribed. It was an operation that had already saved the lives of women with less restrictive insurance policies. Every day, there are Americans whose illnesses lead to serious complications or death simply because they could not afford timely and appropriate health care. How does society morally justify the existence of a health care system like ours — that excludes some people from vitally necessary protections that are available to others?

After Kurt and Peg H. had been swept from affluence into bankruptcy, *NBC Today* reported the story: a gap in their health insurance coverage left the couple unprotected from $300,000 in medical bills for treating their son's leukemia. Every day, middle-class American families are struck by financial calamity because of gaps or loopholes in their health insurance. How does society justify the existence of a health care system like ours — so costly that it bankrupts some of the families who use it?

The Associated Press reported that twenty-one other countries, including Singapore, have lower infant mortality rates than the United States. Every day in America, babies are born without much chance of living through their first year solely because their mothers never had prenatal care. How does society justify a health care system like ours—that makes preventive care so expensive that many citizens are condemned to suffer life-threatening conditions that could have been avoided?

Those are some of the questions we Americans are forced to ask ourselves as we view the condition of our health care system.

The only possible moral justification would be necessity: that economic necessity requires care to be denied to some so that others—who are somehow more worth saving—might live; that there simply is no way to deliver high-quality care at prices families can afford; that there just isn't enough money available for preventive care; that it is politically impossible for a democracy to make high-quality care affordable for all; or that it is simply beyond the organizational skills of human beings to do a better or more equitable job of delivering health care.

It is in this context that we view the health care system just next door, in the country Americans believe to be most like our own. If there is one lesson we must seek, it is this: not *how* to reform our health care financing, but simply *whether* we can any longer find moral justification for delaying reform.

The authors of *Looking North for Health* present a powerful case that it is clearly possible for a Western democracy much like our own to deliver comprehensive, high-quality health care in an affordable way to everybody in the country. The proof is Canadian health care, a North American health system that works. What they show us is a system that, like ours, has flaws and shortcomings but that, unlike ours, provides high-quality care for nearly everybody, controls costs so that high-quality care remains affordable, and has mechanisms that make it responsive to the public will.

The successes of the Canadian system, documented in this book, may or may not provide a blueprint for reform in the United States. But they clearly do present us with a moral imperative for action.

Looking North for Health provides a multifaceted portrait of Canadian health care, viewed from a range of perspectives, including those of patient, doctor and hospital, elected government official, provincial bureaucrat, business executive, and scholar. We examine the scope of the Canadian system from coast to coast—and within the "two solitudes" of francophone and anglophone societies. We examine the continuum of care from acute to chronic that gives meaning to the Canadian promise of comprehensiveness.

For many Americans, reading this book will involve some culture shock. Our assumptions about what is or is not possible are challenged, not by theory, but by the everyday reality in Vancouver and Edmonton and Ottawa. The assumption that greater government involvement in health care financing must mean less autonomy for doctors is challenged by the reality that Dr. Allan S. Detsky describes in Chapter Three, a reality that includes a greater degree of physician autonomy than insurance companies allow doctors in the United States. The assumption that universal, comprehensive health care will obviously cost more than a system that limits coverage is challenged by the reality that health care costs Canadians far less than Americans are paying.

One assumption about health care financing played a key role in the creation of this book. I was spending an afternoon talking about the politics and economics of reform with an outstanding reporter in Washington, Bob Rosenblatt of the *Los Angeles Times,* who—as he is inclined to—was asking difficult questions. Bob understood that Canada's provinces run their health plans on global budgets, setting fixed total amounts of money in advance to cover the year's health bills—and pay their hospitals on the same annual lump-sum basis. What happens, he asked, when a health system or a hospital that is on a global budget runs through the annual budget a month before the year ends? Does that force a shutdown in medical services? Doesn't the threat of running short force rationing all year long?

Canada's provincial health plans do utilize global budgets, but for some reason, shutdowns in various provinces every late November or early December don't seem to occur. Still, wasn't rationing inevitable, as Bob implied? After all, we seemed to have elements of rationing here in the United States: emergency rooms shutting down in city after city, older Americans leaving prescriptions unfilled because of cost, more and more middle-class families postponing visits to the doctor because insurance no longer covered enough of the doctor's fee. Did they have rationing in Canada, too?

The dean of the Washington health press corps, Spencer Rich of the *Washington Post,* raised the same question later that week. I still didn't have a good answer.

It was a problem for me because the drive for health care reform was beginning to pick up steam and the consumer group I work for, Families USA Foundation, was in the middle of the growing national debate. If there were good ideas in Canada, we at Families USA should be spotlighting them, especially because two special interest groups trying to block comprehensive reform — the American Medical Association and the health insurance industry — were taking potshots at the Canadians, accusing them of denying high-tech medicine to patients.

If health beat reporters as seasoned as Rosenblatt and Rich didn't understand the Canadian system, who in the press corps did? It didn't seem right to let the insurance industry version of reality prevail unchallenged. That's how we at Families USA came to organize a forum for the press on Canadian health care in the fall of 1989.

With the help of Senator Jay Rockefeller, who was then chairing the Pepper Commission's deliberations on the future of American health care and long term care, we arranged a forum on Capitol Hill. We invited Senate and House legislative aides working on health care as well as the health beat reporters of the national press.

Two officers of the Canadian Embassy, Norman London and Gail Tyerman, gave us a great deal of help in reaching top-flight Canadian health experts to speak at the forum, starting with the Tory cabinet minister who then headed the Canadian health care system, Perrin Beatty, minister of National Health and Welfare. (The fact that Beatty had moved from defense minister to health minister provoked culture shock in Washington, especially because he was being described by the Canadians as a political leader on the rise. But the Canadian health minister's budget is much larger than the defense minister's, and health is a much higher-profile post than defense in Ottawa.) The minister's speech at that Capitol Hill press forum appears as Chapter Two.

The forum was a success by most measures. But it didn't succeed in convincing Bob Rosenblatt or Spencer Rich that global budgets wouldn't by definition require rationing. After all, they continued to ask, what will happen when the annual budget runs out on the first of December? We Americans tend to think of our way as reality and other ways as hypothetical. We tend to ask what it would be like *if* we were to do it differently, rather than what it is like where it *is* done differently.

As Americans debate the future of our health care system, examining all of the woulds and might-be's, *Looking North for Health* is about what is really happening in fact, not theory, just north of us.

Audience

Despite the openness of the world's longest unarmed border, and the fact that New Yorkers and Californians live a lot closer to Canada than to each other, Americans still don't know much about our northern neighbors — or their health care system. And that extends to many of us who really should: health reporters, legislators, policy analysts, health care activists, physicians, nurses, hospital administrators — everyone, in fact, who is troubled about where we are and concerned about where we should go.

That's the reason *Looking North for Health* has been written in nontechnical language. We sought to achieve accessibility as well as accuracy throughout the book. This book has been written not just for health policy professionals and students of Canadian affairs, although the book should prove valuable to them, but for everybody who is, or wants to be, involved in the national debate on the reshaping of American health care. It has been written so that the debate can be informed by an accurate and comprehensive understanding of the experiences of our closest neighbors.

Misinformation breeds in an atmosphere of inadequate

information. The *National Review,* for example, warned its readers of the dangers of Canadian-style health care. The wait for a mammogram in Newfoundland is two and a half months, according to the *National Review.* The truth is, however, that in that remote, relatively poor, and sparsely populated province, the wait is about two and a half *days,* not months, and there is no wait at all in emergencies.

At a recent West Coast conference on health care, one speaker explained that Canada's success demonstrates the value of using medical copayments in designing a system. The speaker, despite his air of confidence, simply didn't know that medical copayments aren't tolerated in Canada.

Looking North for Health was written to fill the rather large information gap about Canadian health care and to suggest lessons we might profitably draw for our own future.

Overview of the Contents

Our book begins with two overviews. The first, in Chapter One, is by Robert G. Evans, Canada's most distinguished health economist, based at the University of British Columbia in Vancouver. This is the only chapter that has previously appeared in print; it is edited from an article in *Daedalus: The Journal of the American Academy of Arts and Sciences.* It sets the cultural and philosophical ground for a discussion of the Canadian health care system, and I think it is a brilliant analysis.

The second overview, in Chapter Two, is by Perrin Beatty. Americans may be surprised at the fervor with which a Tory defends national health insurance, but the fact is that every one of Canada's major parties is solidly committed to the enormously popular system, from the ultra-right Social Creditists to the social democratic New Democrats, who first crafted the system. But Beatty's fervor goes beyond political survival; still a young man, he was raised under the umbrella of Canadian health, and he shares the widespread pride in a system that works better than the system used by Canada's powerful neighbor to the south. His comments include some impromptu remarks that allow Americans to get a flavor of how strange *our* system looks to the outsider. Challenged by articles in U.S. newspapers that questioned the Canadian refusal to allow people to, in effect, *buy* their way ahead of other people in line, or *buy* better health care than others get, Beatty expresses his personal discomfort with the un-Canadian notion that "someone could jump the line as a result of having money."

Chapter Three, written by a distinguished Washington journalist, Jerry R. Estill, presents several perspectives on the system. Physician Allan S. Detsky and hospital administrator W. Vickery Stoughton allow the reader to see what health care looks like to the patients who use the system and the doctors and hospital administrators who work in it. Detsky is an internist and, like most internists, has been trained to carefully observe and listen to his patients. Unlike most internists, he is also a health economist with a doctorate from MIT to match his medical degree from Harvard. While American trained, he is a Canadian and his values reflect it. His description of the system goes a long way toward explaining why more doctors immigrate to Canada than emigrate, despite the unconstrained fees available south of the 49th parallel.

Stoughton, on the other hand, is an American who has headed hospitals in both countries. A former CEO of Duke Medical Center in North Carolina, he presided over the consolidation of The Toronto Hospital, a sprawling complex of medical institutions in the Ontario metropolis. Having held such prestigious and responsibility-laden posts in major medical centers on both sides of the border, he brings a unique point of view to the discussion. His experiences include dealing firsthand with provincial bureaucrats in shaping his hospital's annual global budgets — and coping with economic stresses on hospitals in the United States.

A third perspective is provided by a Canadian who has worked as a business executive on both sides of the border. Retired from the vice presidency of Chrysler Canada, William J. Fisher has conducted contract negotiations with the United Auto Workers in Michigan and the Canadian Auto Workers in Ontario. His comments on the economic realities square with what most Chrysler executives, including Lee Iacocca, say. Fisher also expresses his personal observation that autoworkers on his side of the border are healthier, because there are no economic disincentives to preventive care.

Just as Detsky portrays the one-on-one contact of doctor and patient, pollster Ian McKinnon views the aggregate of Canadian attitudes about the system, grounded in their contact with the system as patient, taxpayer, and voter. McKinnon, who now serves in the British Columbia bureaucracy, was a pollster for the ruling Conservative government in the last federal elections. He notes in Chapter Four that the broad attitudinal gap between Canadians and Americans on health care is rooted in the very different realities on the two sides of the border. One of the key questions American pollsters ask—"How concerned are you about your ability to afford health care for your family?"—can't be asked in Canada, because nobody there understands the question.

One argument that Evans makes in Chapter One is challenged quite convincingly by McKinnon in Chapter Four. Evans sees the differences between the U.S. and Canadian health care systems as expressing fundamental differences in how Canadians and Americans view the role of government. As a public opinion analyst, McKinnon thinks that the causal relationship flows in the opposite direction: Canadians and Americans view their governments differently because of the different health care systems. Governments that deliver the goods earn trust; governments that allow essential services to become unaffordable don't.

Chapter Five, by former Saskatchewan premier Allan E. Blakeney, offers a personal political history of "how it all got started." Often called "the Father of Canadian Health Care," Blakeney was in at the beginning: the 1960 provincial election in Saskatchewan, the doctors' strike in that prairie province, and the creation of the first public health insurance anywhere in Canada. Based on extensive personal insight, Blakeney talks about the nitty-gritty of the political struggle. To U.S. politicians and health care activists looking toward major political struggles here, this may prove to be the most instructive chapter.

Chapters Six and Seven—by Rosalie A. Kane and Paul Pallan, respectively—look at the Canadian long term care systems. While there has been too little information about Canadian acute health care available in the United States in the last few years, there has been virtually none at all about Canadian chronic care. That's a shame, especially because some of the most exciting advances Canada has made in organizing the delivery and financing of care have been precisely in the field of long term care.

What sense is there in helping someone with heart disease — as our Medicare does — but not helping someone with Alzheimer's disease? The Canadians understand that comprehensive care must include the entire continuum of care: preventive, acute, and chronic care, as well as physician, skilled nursing, and custodial care. If a health condition temporarily or permanently deprives a person of the full ability to carry on normal daily activities — bathing, dressing oneself, preparing food, eating, using the toilet, or getting about — that person needs help every bit as much as somebody whose health condition requires medical treatment. Indeed, as the British Columbians working in Paul Pallan's Continuing Care program have learned, the two problem areas are intertwined in real life. Ignoring long term care drives up the costs, and drives down the value, of providing acute care.

The final section of the book draws conclusions about the Canadian system — in Chapter Eight, by Orvill Adams — and the lessons we can learn from it — in Chapter Nine, by Ron Pollack.

Orvill Adams, formerly chief economist for the Canadian Medical Association (their version of the American Medical Association) and coeditor of this book, gives us a look at how the system as a whole functions. Toward the end of his chapter, he provides a concise answer to reporter Rosenblatt's questions — the questions that really got this book started one spring afternoon in 1989: what actually happens when the lump-sum annual global budget is expended before the year ends? Does that force a shutdown in medical services? Doesn't the threat of running short force rationing all year long?

While recognizing that there have been short-term planning gaps in Canada from time to time, Adams argues that the answers to Rosenblatt's questions are: nothing serious, no, and no.

Clearly, there are lessons to be learned from Canada; Ron Pollack sketches out eleven of them. Pollack, a former law school dean who is the executive director of Families USA Foundation, is an American deeply engaged in the debate over health care financing. He argues that a reformed health care financing system might not look exactly like the Canadian model, but that it must be based on a notion Canadians have come to understand: comprehensiveness, universality, and cost-effectiveness are not menu choices among which one may pick and choose. Achieving any one requires the achievement of all three.

Acknowledgments

Jerry R. Estill made a major contribution to the editing of this entire book. Without his efforts, the book might never have been completed. Also helpful in putting the book together were Janice Gault, Tamara Lyn, Katie Richards, Gail Ross, Barbara Campbell, and Aviva Shlensky, all of whom have my gratitude.

Washington, D.C.   Arnold Bennett
December 1992

The Editors

Arnold Bennett is media director of Families USA Foundation, a nonprofit group based in Washington that advocates for national health care reform, for a long term care social insurance system, and for the income security of the vulnerable elderly and their families. He is a former media consultant who worked on behalf of progressive congressional candidates in sixteen states and on several presidential campaigns. He has also served as a consultant to the Department of Labor on worker health education, as well as to the AFL-CIO Office of Occupational Safety and Health, the Workers' Institute for Safety and Health, and a number of labor unions. He has advised numerous members of the United States Senate and House of Representatives regarding American attitudes toward health care. As a filmmaker, Bennett has been associated with a number of highly acclaimed works as producer, director, and writer. His *Books Under Fire,* a documentary about censorship, was nominated for an Emmy in 1982. His films have won awards at film festivals in New York, Chicago, Washington, Alabama, and Switzerland.

Orvill Adams is a principal in Curry Adams & Associates, a health policy and health, education, and social services planning consultant organization based in Ottawa. The group has clients worldwide. Adams also works with the World Health Organization of the United Nations in health care development. Prior to founding Curry Adams, he was director of economic research and policy analysis at the Canadian Medical Association for ten years. His duties included preparing and presenting briefs to Parliamentary and Senate committees and overseeing studies on the financing, organization, and management of the Canadian health care system. Adams previously was acting director of research for the Association of Canadian Medical Colleges and a researcher and analyst for the Ottawa-Carleton Regional District Health Council Planning Program.

The Authors

Perrin Beatty is the Minister of Communications of Canada. He formerly served as Minister of National Health and Welfare and also served as Minister of National Defense, Solicitor General, Minister of National Revenue, Minister Responsible for the Canada Post Corporation, and Minister of State for the Treasury Board.

Allan E. Blakeney is a visiting scholar at the University of Saskatchewan College of Law. He was elected to the Saskatchewan legislature in 1960 and reelected in successive elections until his retirement in 1988. He was the premier of Saskatchewan from 1971 to 1982. Blakeney holds degrees from Dalhousie University and from Oxford, where he was a Rhodes Scholar.

Jerry R. Estill is a Washington-based writer and editor who has written extensively about medicine, health policy, and politics during a twenty-five-year career as a daily journalist.

Robert G. Evans is professor of economics at the University of British Columbia. He is also a National Health Research Scientist and fellow of the Canadian Institute for advanced Research.

Rosalie A. Kane is a professor at the School of Public Health at the University of Minnesota. She was editor-in-chief of the *Gerontologist* from 1989 to 1992. She is a prolific author and acts as a consultant to numerous federal, state, and private groups. Her research emphasizes long term care programs and policies. She is coauthor of *A Will and a Way: What the United States Can Learn from Canada About Caring for the Elderly* (1985).

Ian McKinnon is Deputy Minister of the British Columbia Ministry of Economic Development, Small Business and Trade. He formerly was Assistant Deputy Minister for the British Columbia Ministry of Finance and Corporate Relations. Prior to entering government service, McKinnon was president and chair of Decima Research, the leading opinion-polling firm to Canada's Conservative Party. He also has served as policy adviser to the Prime Minister of Canada.

Paul Pallan is Assistant Deputy Minister of the Royal Commission — Strategic Development, British Columbia Ministry of Health. He previously served as executive director of the Continuing Care Division of the Ministry of Health and Ministry Responsible for Seniors and as executive coordinator for the provincial Office for Seniors.

Ron Pollack is executive director of Families USA Foundation. He formerly was dean of the Antioch University School of Law and was founding director of the Food Research and Action Center. Pollack often testifies before Congress and is a frequent guest on radio and television programs focusing on health and long term care. He served as a health policy adviser to the Clinton transition team.

Looking North for Health

Dear Editor:

I have read all about the health care plans in the paper. I have done a little work to find out what the general public Canadians think about their health plan. Everytime I see a car with Canadian license plates, I go up and talk to them. They are all nice to talk with, and I ask them how they like their health care plan. So far, 99% of the Canadians I've talked to like their system. They say it is such a peace of mind and the service at the doctor's office and hospitals is really quite good.

If the ordinary run of the people like it, that's all we need to know.

—Ove Madsen, Glendive,
in a letter to the editor of the
Montana Senior Voice

CHAPTER 1

Health Care in the Canadian Community

Robert G. Evans

The "scientific" understanding of human health and illness—the collection of life sciences and associated technologies that generate the intellectual bases for clinical activity—is an international cultural enterprise. Differences among nations are at most different accents in a common language. Patterns of medical practice, "who does what and how and to whom," may vary internationally depending on where a new drug, technique, or piece of equipment happens to have been developed first. But diffusion, like treason, is largely a matter of dates.

The provision of health services, the application of this common intellectual property, is carried out by trained individuals and within organizations that are also quite similar, throughout the industrialized world at least. Physicians, hospitals, nurses, pharmacies, and dentists are virtually universal features of the international health care landscape, although their definitions and competencies may vary in detail. But their patterns of work and their interrelationships are more diverse, being powerfully influenced by the specifics of each national reimbursement system—the set of institutions and processes whereby financial resources are assembled from the general population and then distributed among the providers of care.

1

This health care "industry" accounts for a very large proportion of economic activity in all modern societies — between 8 and 12 percent of nation income.[1] Each country has evolved a distinctive way of organizing, and especially of paying for, its provision of health services. Through these systems, societies show their individuality. Thus, the Canadian health care system, as distinct from the Swedish, or the American, or the British, is a particular way of structuring organization and payment rather than a type of medical knowledge or practice.

Each nation is both legatee and prisoner of its own history and its enduring cultural values and symbols. Students of comparative health care systems emphasize the fundamental continuity of institutions, despite occasional announcements of radical reform and the continuing background rhetoric of rapid change. When "revolutions" occur — the creation of the National Health Service in the United Kingdom, for example, and of the universal public health insurance plans in Canada — they turn out on close examination to have deep historical roots and to represent the continuation of old traditions under new names.[2]

This underlying stability reflects the fact that a nation's health care system is a massive and complex social undertaking, not to be tampered with lightly. The system in place at any moment balances a multitude of conflicting interests and objectives, both overt and covert. But it also serves as a symbol of the fundamental shared values of the society.

Health care is perceived (not always accurately) as a matter of life and death. Access to care may determine the very continuation or termination of the individual, a matter in which the community as a whole is deeply concerned. More generally, the health of an individual is regarded in most societies as a precondition of full participation in the life of the community, like legal or political status, and not merely as a "commodity" of purely private interest.

The financing of health care thus serves as a mirror or a lens in which those dominant cultural values can be viewed and compared from one society to another. The comparison between Canada and the United States is particularly instructive. These very similar societies with very similar systems of medical care have developed radically different funding systems. The behavior and subsequently the organization and performance of the two systems have increasingly diverged in response to markedly different financial opportunities and constraints.[3]

For the student of health care systems, the interesting question is how various financing systems have influenced system behavior and organization. The deeper and more difficult question is why the two societies have evolved such radically different ways of funding health care. The first is a generic question about the behavior of health care systems; the second is a specific question about Canadian, and American, society.

For the differences *did* evolve. They were not, like the parliamentary and presidential systems of government, matters of inheritance. Modern systems of health care finance are a response to technical and social pressures that developed in the twentieth century, and it is within the last forty years that the Canadian and American roads have diverged so sharply. The public systems of hospital insurance were put in place in each of the Canadian provinces between 1946 and 1961 and the medical insurance systems between 1962 and 1971. Supporting federal legislation and cost sharing were added in 1957 and 1966 (effective 1968), respectively. The American system took on its modern form in 1965.[4]

Thus, English-speaking Canadians who seize on their health care system as one outstanding illustration of a rather elusive cultural identity ("Are we *really* different from the Americans?" they ask) have got it right. The Canadian approach to funding health care may be markedly superior to the American on various objective and widely held criteria — many students of health care, including this one, believe that it is — and if so, the Canadian system is an important and rather rare collective achievement. Like beating the Russians at hockey, beating the Americans at anything is a source of considerable satisfaction.

The more basic point is simply that the Canadian health care system, precisely because it *is* different, responds to and reflects significant, if perhaps subtle, features of "Canadianness." It is one of the most convincing forms of evidence, perhaps *the* most convincing, that we are not Americans after all. (It may be difficult for non-Canadians, whether Americans or others, to appreciate what a relief that is.) But our approach differs from the various European health care systems as well, although we are closer to Europe than to the United States, and again the differences are indicative of underlying cultural values.

To fully describe the health care funding and delivery system of each Canadian province would be a mammoth undertaking interesting only to the most dedicated specialist. Each province is different, and the picture is constantly changing in detail. Nor are the details unimportant. There are significant differences in system behavior from one province to another and over time. Analysts who insist that "the Canadian system" is not one but ten (twelve, if one counts the territories) are right.

The User's Perspective

But those who perceive a well-defined common pattern within the diversity are not wrong either. From the point of view of the ordinary Canadian citizen playing the various roles of potential or actual patient, of taxpayer, and of voter, the form of organization and payment is essentially similar across all the provinces. Moreover, from the user's perspective, the system has remained more or less stable for about twenty years. The major conflicts and changes of this period have deeply concerned providers and governments at both the federal and the provincial level but, with few exceptions, have not directly affected the ordinary citizen as he, or more often she, has used and paid for health care.

That Canadian in the street, confronted with what she believes to be a health problem, may decide to consult a physician. She will normally go to a general practitioner in independent private practice (though she may approach any physician she chooses), and the physician may or may not accept her as a patient. Free choice of physician — and patient — is an established principle.

When the patient arrives, the physician will do the sorts of things physicians do — taking a history and noting the symptoms; performing, prescribing, or recommending various diagnostic and therapeutic maneuvers, drugs, or further consultations; and if the condition warrants, sending the patient to a hospital at which the doctor has admitting privileges. Almost any specialist consulted will also be a private practitioner, having a close association with one or more hospitals but not usually being a hospital employee. At no point will there be any charges to the patient for the services of the physician or the hospital, although obviously there are both monetary and nonmonetary costs involved in seeking and receiving care.

(All generalizations, including those in this chapter, are false. There will be charges for services that are judged "medically unnecessary"; in some provinces, such charges include self-referral to a specialist. Private hospital accommodation that is not in the physician's opinion required by the patient's condition may be had on payment of a "preferred accommodation differential." Elective cosmetic surgery is likewise chargeable to the patient. Finally, prescription drugs outside the hospital and dentistry are not covered under the universal hospital and medical insurance plans. Individual provinces have prescription drug and dental insurance plans, but these usually cover only part of the population and/or part of the outlay.)

Reimbursement

The physicians will be reimbursed for their services by an agency of the provincial ministry of health, according to a uniform schedule of fees negotiated at periodic intervals by that agency and the provincial medical association. With minor exceptions, however, the decisions about which services to provide or recommend are entirely up to each physician and subject to the compliance of the patient.

Claims for reimbursement are checked to make sure they conform to the rules for payment included as part of the negotiated fee schedule in force. In addition, "practitioner profiles" are screened to identify patterns of practice that are extremely unusual relative to norms defined by the behavior of a physician's peer group — but these are very wide bounds. In general, the clinical autonomy of the physician is maintained.

The hospital, however, will not be reimbursed directly for the particular services provided to this patient. Hospitals are supported through global budgets negotiated annually with the ministry of health. Salaries of physicians employed by the hospital—residents and interns, salaried chiefs of service, emergency room staff—are paid from the global budget. Diagnostic services and prescription drugs provided to inpatients are likewise included, but diagnostic services provided to ambulatory patients, by either hospitals or freestanding facilities, may be paid for through fees for individual services.

The hospital and medical services are thus almost entirely (between 90 and 95 percent) reimbursed from government budgets. The overall share of public funding for health care is substantially lower—about 75 percent—because expenditures for dental care and nonprescription drugs, and a significant share of those for prescription drugs, are met through direct patient payment or private insurance.

There is also substantial direct payment for long term institutional care, although the public-private split here is largely a matter of bookkeeping. Patients in extended care hospital beds and publicly supported residents in other long term care facilities are charged a per diem fee, calculated not on the basis of the actual charges but as a share of the minimum public pension. The logic of this charge is that the few patients who are in such care (and who now account for a large, and growing, share of hospital days) are in effect being provided with room and board by the hospital. Since the public pension is also intended to provide a minimum standard of living, there is no obvious justification for the state to pay twice. But insofar as this component of private payment represents absorption of another form of public support, its privateness is more form than substance.

Funding

From general taxation and federal grants, provincial ministries of health raise the revenue to support the health system, which is their largest single activity. In the beginning, these grants were proportional to the provinical outlays on medical and hospital care, but since 1977, they have been set by formulas unrelated to actual outlays. Accordingly, while a high proportion of health expenditures is actually funded through federal taxation, provincial governments are entirely at risk for any increases in costs (and are the fiscal beneficiaries of cost containment).

Two provinces retain a system of "health insurance premiums," but these are insurance premiums in name only. They are uniform charges unrelated to the risk faced by the person covered or to the overall cost of services. They are de facto compulsory for most of the population, and most important, no one can be denied services for failure to pay. The uninsured resident who uses services may be billed for back premiums but not for the cost of the services. (In the same way, the property owner who has not paid municipal taxes will be billed for back taxes but will not be denied the services of the fire or police departments upon need and will not be billed for the actual costs of the services received.) Accordingly, these premiums are treated by all analysts as part of the general tax system, not as a separate "insurance" system.

Stripped of a vast array of fascinating detail, the Canadian health care system is a fully linked triangular relationship. Members of the public receive care "free" as patients and pay for it through the general tax system. Professional providers determine the appropriate care to be provided to patients, unencumbered by any considerations of what the patient is able or willing to pay for, and are reimbursed in forms and at rates determined in negotiation with provincial governments. Those governments, in turn, raise the necessary revenues through taxation and distribute them to providers.

This picture is incomplete, however, in that it presupposes a health care system with a fixed capacity, a given labor supply, and facilities such as hospital beds and equipment. But physicians cannot admit patients to beds that do not exist, or refer them for diagnostic or treatment services that are not available. Nor can patients be seen by physicians who have not been trained. The reimbursement system must cover not only the cost of current operations but also the costs of reproducing, expanding, and upgrading the existing system. These capital costs, in the broadest sense, include new technology — equipment and techniques and the financing to support them — as well as the construction of new hospital capacity and the training of additional professionals to direct its use.

The flow of capital into the health care sector and the determination of the amount and type of service it will offer is also negotiated by the professional community and the provincial governments, partly directly and partly through political pressure.

Negotiation of capacity reflects the overlap between two different bases for public decision making, both generally accepted as legitimate and thus a source of conflict. The professional community is believed to have special expertise in deciding what services are required to meet the needs of the population served. In each medical case, the provider determines what is medically necessary — that is, what clinical interventions are appropriate in the care of the patient. Clinical autonomy at the level of the individual, then, logically extends to questions of what types and amounts of facilities and personnel should be available to meet the needs of patients collectively.

The provincial government has an equally legitimate role, however, in deciding what to pay for, where, and when, so long as it acts (and in this field it does) with broadly based public support. This right to make legitimate choices among medical and nonmedical priorities on the community's behalf is further strengthened by the fact that, as a matter of common observation, the skills and knowledge acquired and deployed in the clinical setting with individual patients do not in general carry over to the epidemiological or planning context. The whole is not simply the sum of the parts.

Nor, as I have indicated, is the practitioner a disinterested interpreter of the community's needs. New facilities translate into expanded practitioner incomes and professional opportunities. Negotiations over access to new capital inevitably respond to provider as well as patient interests.

These formal and informal negotiations, over both current reimbursement and expansion of system capacity, take place almost entirely between providers of care and governments. The public is involved in the negotiations as voters, appealed to by providers as potential patients — to support campaigns for more services — or by governments as taxpayers interested in containing overall outlays. But the system of funding does not allow for separate financial arrangements between providers and individual patients with respect to services covered by the public plan.

Physicians cannot "extra-bill" their patients by demanding additional payments above the negotiated fee schedule payable by the provincial government in return for covered services. (Services deemed not medically necessary, on the other hand, are to be charged to the patient in full, at any amount the physician chooses, in principle. In practice, these turn out to be rather rare.) Looked at from the other side of the coin, patients cannot offer physicians side payments for more favorable consideration.

In some provinces, physicians have the option of simply not participating in the public plan, in which case neither they nor their patients are reimbursed. They may then charge whatever they like for their services. But they cannot work both sides of the street, seeing some patients and/or conditions privately and setting their own fees, and yet also seeing others under the public plan. Furthermore, no private insurer can sell coverage for services already covered under the public plans, and so nonparticipating physicians must make their entire practice from uninsured, self-paying patients. Not surprisingly, few practitioners make this choice.

The economic link between use of care and contribution to its cost has been disconnected through the public programs. The surrounding regulatory structure makes attempts by either providers or patients to reconnect that linkage difficult or impossible — and is intended to do so.

Underlying Values

This balance of rights and responsibilties among individuals, the community, and providers of care reflects the attitudes and values of the Canadian population. It would be naive to imagine that many Canadians had actually thought through in any coherent way the system of values of which their health care system is the concrete expression, let alone that they would all agree. But the level of public support for the present system is extremely high. The system has successfully withstood challenges to its basic principles from several quarters — from medical associations, some provincial governments, and the private insurance industry — and continues to hold off such challenges, because most members of the population approve of it. They believe it works and that it is "right."

At the most basic level, the public funding system embodies a view of the relationship between the individual and the environment. Illness or injury can strike anyone. There is no moral reason why the victim should be exposed to financial insult on top of physical injury. Health care in Canada is free, because to charge the patient is to tax the sick.

Indeed, even if the victim *did* contribute to his or her own misfortune — as the smoker with lung cancer or the teenage motorist has — risk taking is not a calculated, voluntary act. Stupidity is as much a natural force as an unanticipated blizzard, and foolish behavior arises in a social context. There may be good reasons for taxing cigarettes and for identifying and penalizing dangerous driving, but charging health care costs to the estate of lung cancer victims or denying them care if they cannot afford to pay is inherently offensive and serves no useful social purpose.

A person holding an alternate view might say that the natural environment provides ample opportunity to look out for oneself. Illness and injury are indicative of avoidable carelessness, correctable incompetence, or even punishable moral turpitude. ("Bad luck" may be evidence of divine displeasure.) People who get into difficulty should therefore bear at least part of the financial consequences, as well as the physical ones. Such a distribution of burdens is fair (why should others bear the cost of an individual's decisions?) and also tends to encourage "better" behavior. Being responsible for one's own acts is a mark of maturity and morally uplifting. It signifies that one takes care and tries to be competent.

The Canadian funding system implicitly rejects the latter view and treats illness as primarily the result of natural or social malevolence rather than personal default. This view in turn is consistent with a deep sense of the powers of the individual in relation to the environment. The system implies a further judgment about the relationship between individual choice and professional authority. When the patient recognizes a problem, she takes it to a professional, who diagnoses it and determines what treatment is medically necessary.

The legislation governing the public plans explicitly identifies medical necessity as the ground for reimbursement. Individuals are not expected to manage care episodes alone but to draw on professional services as they see fit. Furthermore, professional providers are assumed to be equipped with both a base of knowledge sufficient to determine what ought to be done and an ethical imperative to ensure that they will do it without undue regard for their own interest — that is, they will act "professionally."

In this context, there is no particular point in involving the patient economically. The typical patient follows the orders of authority, and that authority acts responsibly in giving orders.

Still another alternative is to take a more activist view and to see the patient, in choosing among providers and the forms of advice given, as manager of his or her own care. This perspective may also include the concern that providers tend to slant their advice in the direction most profitable to themselves unless monitored by vigilant patients protecting their own economic interests. There may be no unambiguously right response to the patient's problem — it is a matter for individual choice — and even if there is, the professional cannot be trusted to recommend it.

This third view underlies the line of argument that has always been of most interest to economists, particularly those who have limited familiarity with the health care field. Patients, they say, should be exposed to some part of the costs of their own health care, whether or not they are wholly or partly responsible for their illnesses (the ethical case gets a little fuzzy here), so that they will either be more careful shoppers for care and/or will keep the professional ambitions or the greed of providers in check.

The Canadian public has accepted, and continues over-whelmingly to support, a system of health care finance whose basic structure implies that, in this domain, individuals are not responsible for their own misfortunes (or at least no useful pur-pose is served by treating them as if they were). Further, the proper response to such misfortunes is to seek and rely on duly accredited professional authority. Such authority can in general be relied on. Presumably, that is what most Canadians believe. And presumably, citizens of nations that have evolved reim-bursement systems that place direct economic burdens on the users of care implicitly take, on balance, a different view.

But that is only the beginning of the story. The collective funding structure implies that the community accepts respon-sibility for ensuring that the individual will have access to needed care. In itself this is not unusual; the collective provision of the preponderance of, if not all, funding for hospital and medical care is universal in the industrialized world.[5] A society that ex-pressed indifference, in principle, to the potential and prevent-able extinction of some of its members could hardly claim to be called a society at all. What is less common is the degree to which, in Canada, this collective responsibility is placed on the shoulders of government and then interpreted as requir-ing not only guaranteed access but access on equal terms and conditions.

"Equal terms and conditions" lies behind both the removal of all direct financial barriers to the public system and the dis-couragement or suppression of private arrangements, so that everyone has access to the same system. "Equality before the health care system" has been established as a political principle similar to "equality before the law."

Other Health Care Systems

Developments in the United Kingdom in 1987 and 1988 illus-trate a still more extreme form of this risk. Strategic behavior may not be limited to providers. An ideologically hostile govern-ment may seek, and certainly is suspected of seeking, to under-mine a popular public program that it does not dare to attack directly. A policy of restricting funding in the public sector is much more acceptable politically if several of one's most influential supporters are already users of the private sector. The maintenance of a constituency in support of a public program is much easier, on the other hand, if everyone has to use that program. Concerns over quality and access find louder voices in support.

Such interactions between the presence of a private alternative and the quality or even viability of a public system are of considerable interest to students of health care systems. They are important questions, and they weigh with some who are in a position to shape policy. But it is doubtful whether these questions are really fundamental to the differences in public attitude between the United Kingdom and Canada. Is the average citizen even aware of these issues? It seems more likely, at least to this observer, that private medicine in the United Kingdom is simply a continuation of the good old British tradition of snobbery and class privilege, which many an earlier generation of immigrants to Canada was glad to leave behind.

In the United Kingdom, most citizens find it right and proper that the "better" class of people should receive their care under more genteel surroundings and pay for the privilege. Yet most Canadians find this opinion offensive. Health care touches the individual so closely — again the perception of life and death — that it is difficult to separate class-specific medicine from the implication that some people's lives are worth more than others'.

Indeed, Canada has a deep-rooted suspicion of class-based systems of any kind. Private schools are a minor part of the educational picture, private universities are nonexistent, and public transportation is all single class, with the exception of the airlines (why?). Canada may not be a classless society, but Canadians are strongly attached to the belief that it is.

Several of the European health care systems also seem to have a class component in their funding, perhaps a remnant of Bismarck's influence. When health insurance was originally provided for the German worker, it was provided by a government under the control of other interests, attempting among other things to undermine the appeal of socialism. Given this objective, there was no obvious reason to include other classes in the program. Furthermore, the European reliance on various forms of payroll tax draws on labor income alone. By relying on general (primarily income and sales) tax revenues, the Canadian system spreads the burden over all income earners.

As the technology of health care has evolved and its potential costs have grown beyond the reach of almost anyone's budget, more and more groups in the European populations have gained some form of insurance. But coverage in many countries remains linked in one way or another to status. The German sickness funds are defined by occupations, with regional funds for those without an occupational base and private coverage for those with the highest incomes. The Dutch compulsory coverage, again, applies only up to a certain income limit. The Belgian funds recruit on a religious basis.

In general, competition for enrollees is limited. Rather, each fund tends to serve a distinct and separate population. Moreover, above some income level, individuals are expected to pay for their own care and/or purchase private insurance, which may be publicly subsidized. All forms of coverage may be regulated and supplemented to ensure universal coverage but not all in the same system or fund.

That both physicians and patients seem to prefer this approach suggests the symbolic importance of special treatment for the upper classes and of direct access to the patient's own resources for the physician. The right to charge some patients directly, even if only a small fraction of them, rather than having to deal with a bureaucracy (whether public or private) seems very important to physicians in all countries.

The bitter battles over extra billing, culminating in the Ontario physicians' strike of 1986, made clear how important such a right is to physicians in Canada. These struggles, which went on for a number of years before and after the enactment of the Canada Health Act of 1984, made equally clear the extent and the depth of the popular opposition to this practice.[6] This conflict drew sharp lines of battle between the majority of physicians in the country and the majority of the population. The population won.

Thus, while Canadian health care shares with European systems the underlying judgment that illness is an unavoidable misfortune, to be remedied by seeking and following professional advice with funding provided entirely or almost entirely through collective mechanisms, it differs in its powerful commitment to the principle that the provision of care and the pattern of funding should be the same for everyone. We are all equal when faced with disease or death, and our institutions reflect that sense of equality.

Origins of the Canadian System

It is no coincidence that the historical origins of the Canadian health care funding system were in the province of Saskatchewan at a time when its population was almost entirely made up of small farmers and people who supported and depended on the farming industry. Weather and world markets, both beyond any control, dictated everyone's fortunes, and everyone went up and down together. The sense of equality before shared adversity that was natural in this environment also seems to have struck a resonant chord in the rest of the country.

The reliance on collective funding through government was a natural response to a communitywide problem. It was also the usual Canadian response to the country's predicament of how to deal with a small population thinly distributed over a large landmass. In the European countries, highly differentiated and concentrated populations made it natural to begin with aggregations intermediate between the individual and the state—with workers' friendly societies or religious organizations. In an earlier and simpler state of medical and administrative technology, such groups were large enough to pool the expenditure risks of their members, and, most important, were linked by an affinity that makes people willing to share their misfortunes and their care.

In Canada, however, the natural focus for collective activity has always been government. As residents of a small country heavily dependent on world markets, flanked on the north by a large hostile wilderness and on the south by a large—and, well, large—neighbor, Canadians have instinctively turned to the state as the instrument of collective purposes. A multiplicity of competing organizations is a luxury we cannot afford.

Nor is private organization and competition accorded the intrinsic value in and for itself that it receives in the United States. In the rhetoric of the business and economic community, which so strongly influences U.S. policy, even a badly functioning private marketplace often appears to be definitionally superior to a well-functioning public agency. Americans seem to accept the form of economic organization as an end in itself, independent of any external performance criteria. This ideology has never put down deep roots in Canada, where both public initiatives and semiprivate regulated monopolies that pursue some version of public purpose (along with private profit) are a tradition older than the country itself.

Accordingly, the collective funding of health care costs takes place through the monopoly suppliers of hospital and medical insurance in their respective regions — the provincial governments. The Canadian system is socialized insurance, not socialized medicine. But the provinces are also the predominant buyers of hospital and medical services from private physicians and hospitals. This has become central to the control of health expenditures, and thus, to the management of health care delivery.

The recognition of this power, a counterweight to their professional authority and a threat to their economic position, lay behind the opposition of physicians to the creation of the universal public plans. Indeed, the subsequent political struggles over extra billing have served to define more clearly the limits of "physician autonomy."

Medical associations have always attempted, in Canada and elsewhere, to extend their claim of special expertise in the clinical setting to include control over the broader questions of how the delivery of medical care should be organized, how physicians should be reimbursed, and how much. In the debates surrounding Medicare, the passage of the Canada Health Act, and the physician strikes in Saskatchewan (1962) and Ontario (1986), these claims to wider political authority were put very explicitly, in direct confrontation with the power of elected governments. The majority of the population decisively rejected these claims.

Yet, at the time the public plans were set up, there was no general public sentiment in favor of limiting physician autonomy. Indeed, the report of the Royal Commission on Health Services (the Hall Commission) expresses the opposite intention, that the public funding system should not interfere with professional independence.[7] What was perhaps not appreciated was the extent to which organized medicine interpreted that independence as depending on, and therefore conferring, special authority over the whole field of health policy.

The advocates of public insurance emphasized instead the manifest inability of private insurers — privately organized competitive forms of collective financing for health care — to cover the entire population. The laws of the marketplace dictate that competitive for-profit insurers, responsible to their shareholders and competing for subscribers, must inevitably exclude those in greatest need and those least able to pay for either insurance or care. In the majority of cases, such persons would then go without or become a charge on the public purse. (European systems built up from several or many funds can maintain universality because the funds are not in competition for enrollees or organized for profit.)

The real options in Canada, or anywhere else, are not public-versus-private forms of collective funding. Private insurance for the whole population is impossible in a competitive marketplace, because insurers cannot cover the poor and the ill and remain competitive. Still less likely is a real choice between individual and collective funding; the patterns of distribution of needs and of economic resources rule out self-payment for the bulk of health care. The only choices, unless a society is prepared simply to accept the exclusion of a significant proportion of its population from the health care system, are universal public coverage or a mixed public and private system, with the public system covering those with the greatest needs and the least resources.

But this mixed approach, so the Hall Commission argued, would be both administratively much more expensive than the other approach and incapable of providing coverage to much of the population, not only on equal terms and conditions but at all. The history of the U.S. system, with the world's highest and most rapidly escalating health care costs, the highest proportion of funds going to administrative costs, and nearly 20 percent of its population uninsured (and perhaps another 10 percent grossly underinsured), bears out the Hall Commission's predictions rather well.

The Canadian Approach

In summary, then, the Canadian health care system reflects a strong commitment to egalitarianism combined with a strong respect for, and substantial confidence in, duly constituted authority. This authority includes both the politically legitimate authority of the state and the professionally legitimate authority of the providers of care. These attitudes stand in sharp contrast to those lying behind the American approach, where the health care funding system, like many other institutions, responds to a combination of individualism and suspicion of authority. But the emphasis on egalitarianism also distinguishes the Canadian approach from those in a number of the European countries, where remnants of class- and status-based funding and care persist.

The reliance on government raises one of the most fundamental questions in Canadian political organization: Which government? The longest and most carefully defended border in the world is between the government of Canada and the governments of each of the provinces. Canadians have a fascination with federal-provincial relations that most other nations reserve for religion or sex.

It is inevitable that the health care funding system as the expression of many of our national symbols and values should provide a setting for playing out federal-provincial conflicts. These, in turn, reflect the extraordinary ambiguity of Canadians' feelings of nationality: Are we really citizens of one country or of ten provinces in a loose association of convenience? Well, it depends. In the particular case of health care, it depends on either creative federalism or constitutional subterfuge, according to one's point of view.

The British North America Act of 1867 — the act of the British Parliament that until 1982 provided the constitutional basis for the government of Canada — specified that matters pertaining to health care were under the jurisdiction of the provincial governments. Such matters were at that time seen as local problems, of no great interest to the national government. The federal government has, accordingly, no constitutional authority to run a health service or a health insurance plan for the general population, and it does neither. Strictly speaking, Canada has no health care system, only a collection of provincial plans.

The federal government does have constitutional authority to raise revenues by direct or indirect taxes and to make grants or other distributions of those revenues. It can make conditional grants to provinces, which can establish and administer public health insurance programs conforming to federally established standards. These standards form the core of Canadian health insurance — public administration, comprehensiveness of benefits, portability between provinces, universality of coverage on equal terms and conditions, and accessibility.

The essential similarity of the provincial plans thus derives from the requirements imposed at the outset as conditions for federal support. That support was initially in the form of cost sharing; the federal government returned to the provinces roughly 50 percent of all outlays on "allowable" health services. An offer of finance on that scale was obviously one that no provinces could refuse. In 1977, the federal contribution was changed to, in effect, a block grant unrelated to actual health care outlays. The contribution remained conditional, but in the new environment the conditions were much more tenuous. In 1984, the federal Canada Health Act made the conditions more explicit and provided for penalties — cash withholding — for provinces whose plans were in default of the federal standards.

No provincial government has ever directly challenged the validity of the basic principles of Medicare — public administration, comprehensiveness, universality, portability, and accessibility. This acceptance reflects their support by a large majority of the populations in each of the provinces. Provincial

governments have argued, rather, that they should have the right
to interpret these general principles on their own initiative. The
role of the federal government should be limited to sending
checks.

On the other hand, it is quite clear that from time to time
provincial administrations have been elected with broad support within the provinces but do not share (or in some cases
even understand) these basic principles. Between the shift to
federal block funding in 1977 and the reassertion of federal standards in 1984 were several provincial initiatives that were hard
to reconcile with these principles. At the same time, public opinion in those provinces remained strongly supportive of Medicare.

In moving to clarify and provide ways of encouraging con-
formity with national standards, the federal government was
both asserting a national interest in this field and acting according to the clearly expressed wishes of its electorate. The federal
Parliament passed the Canada Health Act unanimously, despite
the opposition of a number of provincial governments. All federal parties were acutely aware of the level of public support;
to be against Medicare would be political suicide.

The ambiguity, however, remains. We do seem to have
a habit of electing governments with conflicting principles and
objectives and of hoping that, between them, they will thrash
out an acceptable compromise in areas of competing jurisdiction.

The political ambiguity is now taking on a legal and constitutional dimension. Since 1982, the role of the courts in resolving conflicts of sovereignty between Canadian governments has
dramatically expanded.

Does the new Constitution of 1982 limit the federal spending power insofar as that spending may intrude into areas of
provincial jurisdiction? Or does the answer depend on the relation between the extent of the intrusion and the objectives of
the measure? Will the courts take a narrow view of their own
role, leaving political questions to the politicians, or will they
expand their legislative activities? To take one example central
to the structure of the Canadian health care system, does the
virtual elimination of the economic relationship between provider

and patient violate some fundamental economic right of either provider or patient, or both?

The U.S. Constitution, for example, is interpreted by the courts as entrenching certain fundamental *economic* rights. The rights to "life, liberty, and the pursuit of happiness" seem for Americans to refer, self-evidently, to the pursuit of money. On the other hand, as Canadians are fond of pointing out, the corresponding fundamental constitutional principle in Canada is the preservation of "peace, order, and good government."

Conflicts between providers and governments are, however, inherent in the structure of the Canadian health care funding system and have been from the beginning. It is easy enough to say that the Canadian system reflects a combination of egalitarianism and respect for authority—but which authority?

Patients bring their problems to the professionals, who decide what is to be done. The sum of their decisions defines the level of activity of the health care system. But independently of these decisions, provincial governments decide, with minor exceptions, what the level of spending on medical and hospital care will be. Hence the chronic and occasionally strident complaint of the medical profession that the system is globally "underfunded."

No government, no society, seems willing to make available sufficient funds to support all the activities that health care providers would like to offer their patients or to supply the incomes that the providers would like to receive. The continuing conflict is partly about who should have the authority to determine the size and shape of the health care system and partly a struggle over income shares, over how much doctors, nurses, and other providers should earn relative to the rest of the population.

The conflict, like that between the federal and the provincial governments, is a genuine one between legitimate forms of authority. No politically responsible government can give a private group the key to the public treasury, particularly a group whose priorities include not only making health policy but writing their own income checks. The electorate has given the Canadian governments a clear mandate to manage the overall level of health care expenditure.

On the other hand, governments have never been given a mandate to determine the content of medical practice. Canadians trust their physicians a good deal more than they trust their politicians on such technical matters, and both groups know it. The Canadian system gives governments control over the reimbursement function, not the delivery of care; it is a public health insurance system, not a public health service.

When the two sources of legitimacy collide and professionals' demands exceed public allocations, how should the issue be resolved? Physicians, or at least their organizations, have consistently argued for resolution through a third principle of legitimacy — consumer sovereignty. If the recommendations of professionals exceed what the legitimately elected and supported government wishes to provide, let individuals register their choices in the "marketplace" — let a private system of payment emerge to pick up the difference. Provincial governments, tired of the constant struggle to limit the growth of health outlays on behalf of a rarely grateful public, often find the same concept tempting.

Yet opponents are quick to point out that the consumer sovereignty principle — the individuals' "right" to spend their own resources as they see fit — has minimal relevance in a marketplace that self-regulating providers control.

In a professionally controlled and publicly regulated market, which is the only form we have or are ever likely to see, consumer sovereignty as an ethical principle loses much of its attraction.[8] It becomes merely a justification for mechanisms whereby professionally determined priorities can override those determined through the public political system, which is exactly why professionals favor it. But the determination of who gets what on the basis of the principle of consumer sovereignty yields results that are inconsistent with the other basic values expressed through the health care system — egalitarianism, collective responsibility, and reliance on professional judgment of medical necessity instead of patients' ability to pay (or to buy private insurance).

What self-governing professions offer the consumer is not a competitive market but "guild-free choice," a sophisticated form of restraint of trade, says Alain Enthoven. He also emphasizes the impossibility, indeed the absurdity, of a "competitive market-place" in specific health services for individual consumers. If genuine competition in health care is possible at all, it can be only among integrated organizations contracting to provide a combination of insurance and care on a capitated basis, as American HMOs do, for example.

Canadians have chosen to leave the resolution of the contradiction between professional priorities and political constraints to negotiation between the two parties. Legitimate sources of authority should be able to work out their differences somehow, without necessarily requiring any clearly defined means of resolving the dispute (such as the courts or gunfire). They should be able to discover, and be guided by, the broader public interest — it is the Canadian way.

A nation's health care financing system is not merely a complicated mechanism for displaying its predominant moral and cultural values. It must also do its basic job, raising the resources necessary to support the provision of an acceptable standard and distribution of health care and contributing to, or at least not getting in the way of, the effective management of that care.

The job of organizing, applying, and paying for medical technology has similar objectives in all countries, even if the criteria for evaluation may differ somewhat. This similarity suggests that comparisons of systems' performance around the world should provide a reasonable basis for evaluation.

Such a discussion must include a clear sense of context. All health care systems are in perpetual crisis. Cycles of media attention rise and fall, but the same issues come up over and over again in each system.

The Canadian approach to funding was declared unworkable by its opponents — physicians and private insurers — in the early 1960s, and the same interest groups have continued to detect imminent collapse right up to the present. The American health care system is well into the third decade of the longest-running cost explosion since the great inflation of the sixteenth century. The British National Health Service is gripped by what appears to be the most bitter of its periodic crises. All over

Europe, governments are struggling to contain the costs in the face of aging populations, advancing technology, and growing professional numbers and ambitions. (Their academic advisers, particularly economists, sometimes suggest that they look to the United States for solutions, which makes about as much sense as looking to the old Soviet Union for advice on organizing grain production or the United Kingdom for ski-jumping coaches.)

Still, individuals often regard their own health care systems as the best in the world.[9] Like confidence in one's own physician, confidence in one's own national way of organizing health care seems to be a natural, and perhaps quite functional, response to uncertainty and incomplete information. It may also reflect the adaptation (and perhaps the contribution) of each system to the underlying cultural values.

Thus, Canadians consider getting sick in the United States as the equivalent of a severe mugging. It has similar economic and physical consequences, and provincial governments have sent medical evacuation flights to rescue their citizens from the U.S. hospital system. In contrast to humane and civilized Canada, Americans are left to die in the streets after their money runs out. Nevertheless, Americans continue to refer to their health care system, whatever its problems may be, as the world's best and, to the astonishment of Canadians, appear to be serious! And Americans would be equally astonished, perhaps with as good reason, to see the attachment of the British to their National Health Service, which in the United States is called a nightmare.

Popular acceptance, therefore, is no basis for discrimination among national systems. What can be compared most readily (though comparing them is by no means easy either) is relative overall costs and the stability of those costs over time. Though it might seem the least important aspect of a health care system — compared with, for example, what that system does to and for its patients — comparative cost performance does interact with issues of equity and access and perhaps of effectiveness.

The connection arises because although there are no clear, or at least operational, criteria for deciding how much is enough for any country to spend on health care, it is clear that continuing escalation of costs relative to national resources is not a sustainable situation. In the last decade, all industrialized countries have come to place a high priority on stabilizing the growth of health care costs in their national systems. A system that fails to do so will be changed — it is simply a question of when — and will go on being changed, in increasingly radical ways, until some degree of stability can be attained.

For nearly two decades, the Canadian health care system has achieved a remarkably good record in both preserving universal access to comprehensive coverage and moderating the growth of health care costs. This performance has been outstanding in comparison with that of the U.S. system, which displays accelerating cost escalation, increasingly radical institutional change, and deteriorating equity. The Canadian performance also looks good in comparison with that of Western Europe — a more demanding comparison.[10] On the whole, the European countries have been much more successful in stabilizing their systems than has the United States but less so than Canada, and concerns about equity and access are starting to emerge in those systems that have never had the same firm foundation of egalitarianism.

A more detailed analysis, however, brings out the falsity of the often-asserted conflict between the overall control of the size of the health care sector and the preservation of access and quality of care. A comparison of the Canadian and the American experience, for which detailed data are readily available, shows that the greatest differences in costs — contained in Canada and exploding in the United States — are in the administration of the payment system and in the inflation of physicians' fees.[11] Canada gets an outstanding bargain on the first, and reasonably good performance on the second. In the United States, both are escalating at an accelerating rate. Neither of these components of health expenditures translates into clinical services for patients. The first is simply system overhead — in the United States, pure waste motion — and the second is the result of a struggle over income shares.[12]

There is also a marked difference in the number and cost of diagnostic and therapeutic maneuvers that the average patient undergoes within hospitals.[13] But since many observers of North American hospital care have long expressed concern about over-treatment in hospitals, and since reduced use of hospitals is a major emphasis of U.S. health policy, the difference in treatment intensity cannot be taken as an a priori indicator of reduced access to effective care in the Canadian system.[14]

The Canadian system is by no means a model of efficiency in any absolute sense. As in every other system, there are wide variations in treatment patterns and costs that have no apparent connection to the underlying needs of the populations served. Much of what is done is ineffective, unnecessary, or unnecessarily costly. But these are not problems peculiar to Canada. While it is true that the funding system provides few, if any, rewards or incentives to providers for efficient performance, the same could be (and has been) said for all other national systems. The organizational problems health care poses are devilishly difficult, and Canada has not found a solution that has escaped everyone else.

We have, however, succeeded in removing the economic barriers to access to high-quality health care for the whole population. At the same time, we have stabilized the overall share of our national income taken up to pay for care, and we have shifted the economic burdens from those who happen to be ill to those who can afford to pay. While people in every country may profess to believe that their own health systems are the best ones, the level of satisfaction of Canadians with their arrangements must be among the highest in the world. To a certain extent, our satisfaction reflects our tendency to be smug about our own decency and moral rectitude, but we do get some reinforcement from external observers.

On the other hand, there is also evidence that the compromise between professional autonomy and public fiscal responsibility, which has been central to the operation of the Canadian system, is starting to fray. Provincial governments are finding that moderating expenditure growth is requiring increasing attention to "utilization control" — service patterns and volumes — rather than simply restraint of fees and of hospitals' global budgets. Even moderate increases in health care costs absorb virtually all the governments' fiscal maneuvering room, simply because health is such a large proportion of provincial budgets.

The provincial governments are trying to put explicit caps on overall outlays, and while these may not directly impinge on the clinical activity of the providers, the caps' indirect effects are becoming stronger. As each funding system moves toward overt recognition that it steers health care practice, the system's managers may have to negotiate more explicit objectives and criteria for system performance with providers.

The challenge for the future may be to find ways to discover and express our collective values with respect to the definition of health itself. What sort of outcomes as opposed to services do we as a community think worth buying? And through what institutional channels, present or projected, do we give expression to those views?

If history is any guide, we will be able to watch these issues debated in an open free-for-all in the United States, thoroughly entangled in a web of competing economic interests. The debate will produce analyses of extraordinary competence and clarity, which will not, however, be decisive for actual policy.

Meanwhile, in Canada we will rely on the responsible authorities to come up with some sort of solution or at least a response. As agents, they are very far from perfect, but they may be the best we've got. In the final analysis, defects and all, the system we have seems to be a remarkably good compromise of quality, affordability, equity, and humanity. Not bad, eh?

CHAPTER 2

A Comparison
of Our Two Systems

The Honorable Perrin Beatty

It's a useful and interesting juxtaposition to go from being minister of National Defense, worried about Canada's security and Canada's sovereignty, to being forced to address some of those questions about what we are defending, what it is that our country believes in, and what we stand for as a nation. It's been a very useful experience.

We're a country that's blessed by geography, by good fortune in terms of natural riches, and certainly by good fortune in terms of who our friends are and who our neighbors are, and this enables us to put resources into an area that is key to improving the quality of life of every Canadian.

Comparisons of Canadian and American systems are always interesting because we're alike and we're not alike. While it's true that we're both democracies and strong allies, our political and our social systems are quite different.

The American literary critic Leslie Fiedler once said that Canadians like to emphasize our differences and Americans, our resemblances.

I hope to emphasize a little bit of both. I believe that we have a strong and a fair system of health care in Canada, one that works well for our country and our people. Our resemblances make aspects of it attractive to the United States, and

28

yet our differences mean that it might not be appropriate for you.

Only you can make this choice. It's not for me to sell Canada's health care system to you. It's for me as a guest in your house to explain our health care system and to leave it to you to make your own choice.

Certainly opinion in the United States is divided over its appropriateness for you. On the one hand, a Harris poll reports that 60 percent of Americans favor adopting the Canadian health care system.[1]

On the other hand, the American Medical Association has published a strongly worded report stating that the Canadian health care system is, in its words, "poorly suited to post-industrial societies with changing human service needs."[2]

Now, I'm not sure that either of these two reflections really represented an understanding of our system when those opinions were ventured. I'd like to tell you about the advantages and pressures of the Canadian health system in the hopes that that will shed a little light on the discussion.

Health care is big business. This is true whether you're talking about the United States, about Canada, or about any other industrialized country.

In Canada, we spend more than $50 billion on health each year. The sector employs 7 percent of our work force, including 57,000 physicians and 250,000 nurses.[3] Health care benefits are available to everyone. Our system has survived and developed over the years to the point where it's now studied closely by other countries.

The key to unlocking Canada's relative success is the fact that good health policy is also good economics. It makes sense once you understand the complexities of health markets for us to have a system of health care that's financed largely in the public sector.

Let me start with the three major attributes that I see in a publicly funded, universal health care system.

- First, it's attractive to consumers because access is virtually unimpeded when they need care.

- Second, it's attractive to providers because they are guaranteed payment.
- Third, it's attractive to business for reasons of cost.

Let me explain briefly each of these advantages. Ninety percent of Canadians recently stated that they like our system. They like it because they're free to choose which doctor they see and are entitled to a full range of services regardless of their level of income.

No one waits to seek care because he or she can't afford it. A sudden illness or an accident is not a financial catastrophe for an individual or for a family, as was the case before comprehensive coverage.

For most people, it works like this. The patient receives the service. The doctor bills the government, and the hospital budget pays for inpatient and outpatient care.

Canadians like this system because it's accessible. In fact, they like it so much that it's the one area where they're prepared to see taxes raised to finance increased services, if those increases are truly necessary.

Let me digress here briefly. One of the advantages of discussions like this is they force someone like me, who has grown up with Canada's health care system in place, to begin to examine our system again and to take a look at things we take for granted in Canada.

I read a range of American publications regularly and was very struck by an article that dealt with Canada's health care system, I believe in the *Chicago Tribune*. It was intriguing to me to see the point they made that one of the advantages of Canada's health care system was that we didn't have families who were devastated financially as a result of unexpected medical bills.

Clearly there is devastation, both emotional and financial, when people in a family end up having to go into a hospital. But they don't have the added burden of having incredible medical care costs added on top of everything else.

What was most interesting to me, though, was a criticism that was made of the Canadian health care system, and it got me thinking again. The criticism was that it's not possible in the Canadian system to buy a better level of service, that all Canadians receive the same quality of service. You can't jump the line or receive special treatment if you're willing to pay more money.

The irony to me was that, having grown up in our system, it never struck me that anybody would feel it was appropriate to buy better service or that someone could jump the line as a result of having money.

In Canada, we believe deeply that just as equal treatment under the law is essential, equality in terms of service for health care is a human entitlement. It's not something that comes to you as a result of your ability to earn money.

The thought that you would have unequal treatment based on an individual's ability to pay was something that was so alien to me in reading it that it forced me to go back and to reexamine, I suppose, the principles of our own system. It made me realize that these principles that we take so much for granted in Canada are not taken for granted everywhere else.

As the system in Canada has grown, so have expectations among Canadians about what it can do for them and for their health. The amazing advances in medical technology and new methods of treating chronic disease have opened up new and expensive options. These new and expensive procedures have produced cost pressures on the system, with limited controls in place for their use.

It's not a pressure that is unique to Canada. All of the industrialized countries face similar pressures, forcing us all to choose methods of allocating scarce resources.

Which is better? In the United States, the pressures are decentralized, and they're diffused by the marketplace. In Canada, suspected failures, especially fatal ones, make instant and dramatic headlines and create political pressures on provincial governments.

Despite these problems, Canadians are passionate supporters of the system. From its very inception, it has enjoyed support from all three of our major political parties. No politician would dare tamper with it.

The recent debate over the free trade agreement showed me that Canada's health system has become part of our national identity. The free trade agreement would, it was argued by some, mean an end to Medicare. Of course, the argument was spurious, and the free trade agreement does not and could not affect our health care system or any of our other social programs.

Canadians, however, reacted overwhelmingly and negatively to any such suggestion. Their response showed that universal health has ceased to be just an issue in Canada. It has become a fundamental social value.

It's easy to understand why the public likes the system. It's free, and it's simple to access. What's more surprising is that doctors and other providers seem to like it as well.

A recent survey of physicians found that nearly two-thirds were satisfied or very satisfied with the practice of Medicare in Canada. They like it because, while government provides the financing, it is very reluctant to interfere with the professional autonomy of health administrators or of doctors.

Hospital administrators in Canada are given a global budget at the beginning of each year to provide an agreed-on package of services. Within this broad budget, they have complete control over the day-to-day allocation of resources, and they are responsible to community boards of trustees, not to some far-flung bureaucracy.

Doctors have the same freedom that they have always had to choose the services they believe are most appropriate for the patients. Most of them act as self-employed businesspeople who submit their bills to the government instead of to hundreds of patients or benefit plans.

Since there's only one payer, bad debts are a thing of the past and bureaucratic red tape is held to a minimum.

I'm not trying to suggest that doctors in Canada are completely content with the system. When it was originally proposed, doctors responded with a twenty-three day strike in Saskatchewan.

More recently, when the Parliament of Canada legislated away extra billing, there was another work interruption, this time in Ontario.

We continue to see in the press, and in other places, a healthy tension between governments and providers of health care. This isn't particularly unusual. In Canada and the United States, there is tension between cost controllers, check writers, and health professionals, but the tension manifests itself in different ways.

When physicians ask for higher pay or are concerned about government controls in Canada, it's standard practice, even expected, that they raise these as political issues. Politicians are lobbied and the media is used extensively to develop the argument.

This leads to a level of discussion in Canada that is very public. We don't see this as a drawback. We think this is precisely where a discussion of this nature belongs. It's only fair that the public be involved, since physicians are asking for a higher level of public funding. They're asking for more of the taxpayers' money.

I've talked about why patients like the system and why doctors tolerate it, but perhaps most interesting of all is the often silent support the system receives from the private sector.

Business was skeptical at the beginning about government getting into the health financing business. The private sector in Canada looks on any government involvement with suspicion. Certainly this was true of private insurers, who argued at the time that they could do it better than government.

Over time, however, it's become clear that a public system could deliver quality care for less than a private system grown topsy-turvy.

As recently as 1971, the United States and Canada spent about the same percentage of gross national product (GNP) on health care, 7.6 percent and 7.4 percent, respectively. By the end of the 1980s, our total health care spending was much lower, at 8.6 percent, than that of the United States, at 11.4 percent.[4]

What's the secret to cost control? There's no simple answer, but part of it is that, unlike the American system, our system doesn't involve hundreds of insurance companies. Problems with double billings or dealings with the uninsured are foreign to Canada.

This means that we save money on administration. How much money? In Canada, we spend 2.5 percent of total health costs on administration. The cost of administration in the United States is more than three times that.[5]

Put another way: If the United States spent the same proportion of its budget as Canada, it could save $21.4 billion each year on administrative costs alone. I believe that's based on 1986 American figures.

The cost advantage is gained from the fact that we have a single paymaster in each province of Canada. It's possible to control many of the inputs, such as how much capital investment in human resources should go to health care or where they should be employed.

Business likes our system not just because it's cheaper, but because the burden of paying for it is spread more fairly. In Canada, health care is paid for by personal taxes, corporate taxes, sales taxes, payroll taxes, and other taxes. All Canadians share in the burden according to their ability to pay, and all Canadians benefit.

So patients like it. Doctors admit privately to liking it, and business, when looking at operating costs, appreciates it.

Has it improved the health of the population? We think it has. At the time we introduced the first element of our plan in the early 1950s, our infant mortality rate was running 40 percent higher than Australia's, 30 percent higher than the United Kingdom's, and 5 percent higher than the United States'. By the early 1970s, after the medical care insurance system was fully in place, our infant mortality rate was identical to Australia's and the United Kingdom's and 10 percent lower than in the United States. Today our infant mortality rates are 30 percent lower than yours and among the lowest in the world, at 7 per 1,000 live births.[6]

When Medicare was introduced, we found that pregnant women started showing up a couple of months earlier for prenatal care than they had previously. I don't pretend that all of the improvements in infant mortality rates are attributable to Medicare, but I believe it is a factor, and it's worth noting that since the introduction of it, our maternal mortality rates have dropped by a third.

I hope I've provided some sense of the way our system works and the advantages it offers consumers, providers, and the private sector. But we've really only looked at half the story. Our system must be judged not only by its strengths and weaknesses to date, but also by how well it can respond to new challenges, such as the aging of our population, the emergence of new diseases such as AIDS, and continuing innovations in technology.

In this respect, our system is far from fully developed. As good as I believe it is, I think it's going to have to improve.

Clearly, one pressure for change in both countries is the level and rate of increase of costs. You spend 11.4 percent of your GNP, and we spend 8.6 percent. While the comparison is in Canada's favor, that's not much comfort for health ministers in Canada, because next to the United States, we have one of the highest levels of per capita spending anywhere in the world.

The two dozen leading industrial nations in the world who make up the Organization for Economic Cooperation and Development (OECD) all have lower or similar health spending-to–GNP ratios as Canada.

Now, add to this the fact that health care budgets are the largest single component of provincial government spending, and you can see why cost containment is an issue that never goes away. We are facing the inevitable gap between the health care to which an industrialized society aspires and what it's prepared to spend. It's a gap all industrialized countries face, and we have much to learn from individual techniques pioneered in the United States, such as HMOs and other innovative delivery methods.

Since one of the strengths of the Canadian system is control of costs, we must work hard and look at imaginative new ways of maintaining that advantage.

A second pressure comes from the fact that sometimes our technological advances outstrip our capacity as a society to deal with them. An example that comes to mind is reproduction. Genetic therapy, in vitro fertilization, and a host of other advances make it possible to do things that we thought were impossible just a few years ago.

This has raised a series of ethical, moral, legal, and eco-

nomic questions that remain to be answered. In this particular
case, the prime minister announced a Royal Commission on
New Reproductive Technologies whose function will be to answer these very difficult and intimate questions.

But in most cases, a royal commission is neither possible
nor appropriate, and so we depend entirely on the cooperation
of the provinces, the providers, and the patients to develop acceptable approaches.

In Canada, progress must be based on consensus, and
building consensus can take time. The downside is that it takes
us longer. The upside is that by the time we get there, the
majority agrees.

If we are to make the best possible use of new technologies, it's clear that we'll have to find faster, better ways of working together in reaching a common understanding of the limits
of technology.

A third pressure we must address is the long-standing issue
of health inequalities. In Canada, as in many other industrialized countries, the poor live shorter and harder lives. Despite
the fact the universal health care program has reduced differences in use between rich and poor, we still see a five-year gap
in life expectancy between rich and poor women and a ten-year
gap for men.

A fourth pressure relates to managing our human resources
more effectively. In the past few months, we've had strikes by
nurses. This drastic action comes from people who are the back-
bone of our system but who feel they've not received the respect
or the attention they deserve. It's shortsighted to train people
to care for others and then not discuss the problems or possible
solutions with them. Nurses must be at the table when advice
is needed or decisions are taken. We need to find better ways
to include our partners more effectively.

The fifth challenge is to find new ways to improve the
quality and not just the length of lives of Canadians. There's
a growing consensus that, at least in the short term, greater improvements in individuals' health status will arise out of life-
style and environmental changes than from new medical techniques or higher levels of care.

I think our publicly funded system is well suited to supporting health promotion. In a public system, a government has the necessary scale and the coverage to balance, for example, whether the health of its citizens is better served by two new intensive care hospital beds or by $1 million annually in advertising to discourage teen smoking.

Beyond this, governments are best able to invest in controls in acid rain or improvements in the water quality of the Great Lakes because the health of the environment can help prevent much more costly problems in the health care systems later on.

Digressing on that, irrespective of the type of health care delivery system we have, dealing with these environmental issues — issues such as acid rain, Great Lakes' water pollution, and a whole range of other environmental problems — has enormous benefits, both human and economic, for both of our countries. It's essential that we work together on that. It's essential for the sake of both of our peoples that we succeed in making real progress in this area.

We can't afford to allow it to slide. We can't pretend that the problems aren't real and immediate today. If we want to see tangible benefits for both countries in terms of the quality of life and the length of life for our people, it's essential that both countries get serious about issues related to pollution and issues related to preventable disease.

For example, we expect that some 35,000 Canadians per year will die of tobacco-related diseases. You can imagine the cost to our health care system in terms of dealing with that. You can imagine the economic costs in terms of forgone earnings and the contribution that's made by those individuals who are incapacitated or whose lives are lost entirely, and you can imagine, most important, the tremendous human suffering that's caused as a result of this preventable disease.

Our emphasis needs to be in heading off disease before it takes place instead of looking for remedial action to take after the disease has struck. That's why it's essential that the public sector in both of our countries be involved in making these fundamental decisions about social priorities and about the allocation of resources.

Simply put, it's easier to reallocate resources when you have only one principal source of financing. In the United States, the organization that has to pay may not be the same one that benefits.

These pressures to manage resources effectively assume an even greater importance and urgency when they're seen in the context of our aging societies.

Canada still has one of the youngest populations in the industrialized world, just behind Japan. A major study of Canada's demography shows that our proportion of elderly will be increasing significantly into the next century.

This shift may force us to reexamine how we care for our seniors. For example, we find more seniors, 8.7 percent of them, in Canadian institutions.[6] This is a higher proportion than most other countries, including the United States. I think we can do better and at the same time assist seniors who wish to maintain their independence at home.

Responding to pressures and concerns such as these will require the input of seniors and seniors' advocates. We need to have a better sense for the seniors' vision of the future, and this is where I see organizations such as the Families USA Foundation and like-minded Canadian groups playing such a vital role.

I started this chapter with the premise that good health policy is good economics as well. I hope I've given some sense of why I believe this to be true. I've only touched on how difficult this can sometimes be.

Canada's publicly financed health care system was built through consensus. Federal and provincial governments had to work out a constitutional compromise. Funders and providers had to agree on a division of responsibilities. It took over forty years to put the program in place. Much controversy surrounded its planning and its implementation, and at times the debate was divisive.

While reaching a national consensus takes time, it's the only way I know to be sure policies are consistent and coherent and can stand the test of time. It took a great deal of compromise and cooperation at the provincial and national levels for us to get where we are today. The challenges I see ahead demand that we develop a similar cooperative spirit at the international level.

For example, technology is not constrained by national boundaries, nor are the health effects of acid rain and pollution. Meeting these challenges demands that we work more closely together.

We've started that process. We'll soon have a Coordinating Office for Health Technology Assessment, which will be able to work together with the Office of Technology Assessment in Washington. It's a good example of how we can work together, but much more is possible. I believe there are many ways in which Canada and the United States can develop new partnerships.

In summary, it's possible to have a system that provides high-quality health care, free of point-of-service charges, without breaking the bank, and Canada has proven this. But as a prominent Canadian health economist recently pointed out, nations do not simply borrow other nations' institutions.

I believe the Canadian system is best placed to meet the future needs of Canadians, but I'm not trying to sell it to you. You have to decide for yourselves what system meets your medical and your financial needs.

The point is that by examining each other's experiences, we can extend the range of perceptions of what's possible. Such learning is, of course, a two-way street, and I hope what I have said will help open up just such a two-way street for Canada and the United States. It's a dialogue that can only be helpful to both of our nations.

CHAPTER 3

From Inside the System:
A Physician, Hospital Administrator, and Business Executive Talk About Their Work in Canada

Jerry R. Estill

The choice is clear for Dr. Allan S. Detsky, an American-trained physician who is one of Canada's most renowned internists: he simply cannot imagine working in the U.S. system.

To Detsky — a hands-on, working doctor as well as a policy expert — the freedom of physicians to practice medicine in the best interests of their patients is unnecessarily restrained by the U.S. system.

"I don't think Canadian physicians would in any way wish to go to the system you have in America, or to the system Canada had before we got our current health care system," says Detsky. "Remember, it's not socialized medicine; it's government provision of health insurance."

W. Vickery Stoughton, whose background as a hospital administrator has placed him in contact with physicians in many different specialties, perceives almost exactly the same thing.

Stoughton is an American who spent eight years in Canada before recently returning to a position in the United States. Like Detsky, he draws his conclusions from firsthand experience with both the U.S. and Canadian systems.

"Canadian doctors who have gone to the United States say doctors in the United States do not enjoy the same kind of freedom of practice in America as they did in Canada," says

Stoughton. "These Canadian physicians have come away with an unfavorable opinion of the United States' system, even though it is richer economically than the Canadian system."

Strikingly, the sentiments of Canadian doctors as perceived by Detsky and Stoughton run 180 degrees counter to a common belief in the United States that the Canadian system imposes a government straightjacket on physicians' ability to practice medicine as they think best.

Aside from being a beneficiary of Canada's health insurance system himself, just as his eighty-nine-year-old father is, Chrysler executive William J. Fisher is keenly aware of the benefits it provides employees of his company, as well as those of Ford and General Motors.

Fisher was with Chrysler in the United States until 1977. Like Detsky and Stoughton, then, his opinions are based on firsthand experience with both health systems.

"Health care complaints from employees and retirees in the Canadian auto industry are few and far between," says Fisher. "In my many years of working in the auto industry in the personnel and human resources areas, we had very few complaints, from either union or nonunion employees, with respect to their health care coverage. The coverage is something that has been there for many years. It's taken for granted that auto workers will receive this benefit, and it's much appreciated by them."

A Physician's Perspective

Allan Detsky believes the lack of consensus about how to improve health care in the United States is rooted in the fact that U.S. society has yet to embrace the underlying concept of the Canadian system: that everyone is entitled to comprehensive health care, including long term care for people of all ages.

Even among many in the United States who accept universal access as a philosophically worthy ideal, there is a skepticism about government control and the prospect of runaway costs that Detsky finds hard to understand, given his conviction that the Canadian government "is very watchful of the bottom line, very conscious of cost control."

But the internist says the most widespread misunderstanding of the Canadian system by most people in the United States, doctors included, has to do with how the system actually works on a day-to-day basis, how doctors deal with their patients. In the following paragraphs, he clarifies some of these misconceptions.

I believe the system is extremely patient-friendly in the sense that patients have total autonomy over their own decision making. It's not like what we perceive the British system to be, with patients having access only to certain practitioners. In Canada, patients have easy access to any practitioner they choose — or any number of practitioners.

A Canadian carries a little card with his or her health insurance number on it and can go to any practitioner anywhere in the country.

It's important to note that approximately 50 percent of Canadian physicians are primary care providers, at the general practitioner or family practice level. Although the overall Canadian physician-to-population ratio is comparable to that in the United States, the large proportion of primary care providers in Canada is in sharp contrast to the proportions in the United States, where more doctors go into specialties.

Canadian patients have extremely easy access to those family doctors, because health care is free at point of use, fully paid by the health insurance system, with no copayments or other fees. Canadians use physician services very frequently and are never presented a bill when they do.

The general practitioners or family doctors are free to refer the patients on to specialists to give opinions, order tests, arrange for hospitalization, or do whatever else they think is medically necessary — after consulting with the patients. The specialists' fees also are fully paid by the central insurance program.

Patients can get a second opinion, or even a third. If they don't like their family doctor, they can switch to another. If they don't like the new one any better, they can switch back. If they don't like the consultant, they can ask for another one. There is no limitation on access to physician services at the individual-patient level.

For patients, there is a sense of security in knowing that they're not going to be wiped out financially by catastrophic health events or even minor health events, which can be catastrophic for some families. The fact that Canadians are free to seek multiple medical opinions is something they like a lot. As you'll hear from pollsters, these freedoms to seek the care they want without financial worry help to make the health care system the most popular publicly administered program in Canada.

Very little control is exerted over patients.

Physicians also enjoy considerable autonomy. They are not required to seek approval from an insurance agency, in this case the government, before they order tests. Insurance agencies do not have to give their approval for hospital admissions, or for any medical procedures. Physicians do not have to fill out any forms after they render services, justifying those services to insurance companies.

A friend who is a general internist in the United States was telling me that if she has an AIDS patient in the hospital, she gets a telephone call every three days from the insurance company: "When are you getting him out? When are you getting him out? When are you getting him out?" In Canada, we have no calls like that.

I asked her to estimate how many hours each day the average physician in her practice spends dealing with getting insurance companies' approvals, and with related administrative hassles. She felt it was approximately an hour a day. In Canada, we don't do any of that at all.

In Canada, at the end of the day there is no filling out of forms to justify a hospitalization. There is no insurance company disallowing charges for hospitalizations after they've taken place. For physicians, as for patients, administration is very simple.

Billing is done via a system where each available physician service has a code number. To see how it works, take me as an example. I'm a general internist. You can imagine the variety of patients I see, yet I probably use, at most, ten codes out of the billing code book to submit my claims. I do it by computer and get paid within two or three months.

The only time we don't get paid is if we happen to bill for something that is clearly not allowed, such as overly frequent daily visits to a patient who is hospitalized. If a patient of mine has been in the hospital more than thirty-five days, I can't charge for visiting him or her every single day. If I happen to make that mistake in submitting my bills, I won't get paid for every visit and there will be a little message on my payment that tells me exactly why I'm not getting paid for every visit I made.

Overall, there's very little administrative hassle, and this brings up an interesting paradox. I believe it is the perception of most Americans that government control leads to less autonomy for individual patients and physicians. But in fact the Canadian system, which is totally government run, leads to considerably more autonomy than the pluralistic, market-oriented system in the United States.

I think most American physicians, and probably most American patients, assume that if a government bureaucracy were to run a health insurance program, it would be like the American Medicare and Medicaid programs you have today. There would be all the associated administrative hassles and the filling out of endless forms. That's just not the way it is in Canada, and I don't think that is because Canadians are any better at running bureaucracies or administering government than Americans are.

Government-run programs need not be as complicated and hostile as they are in America. It would be cheaper to have them less complicated and less hostile.

Detsky was born and reared in Canada but spent eleven years in Boston, where he attended medical school at Harvard and served a two-year residency at Massachusetts General Hospital. The vast majority of all physicians now active in Canada graduated from medical school after the introduction of Medicare and have become accustomed to practicing in the system.

"My perception is that the idea of Canadian physicians actually dealing with the pluralistic private enterprise financing system you have in the United States would be untenable," says Detsky. "We couldn't function."

Nonetheless, he says Canadian physicians raise health care questions in the media, much as opposition parties raise them in the legislature. "There's a certain amount of posturing that takes place for purposes of political positioning."

Detsky says one key to the broad acceptance of the Canadian system among its doctors is that payments to primary care providers are significantly higher in Canada than in the United States. "At the top end of the scale, thoracic surgeons in Canada may be making a lot less than their American counterparts, but Canadian family doctors and general internists will be making substantially more than those in America," he says. "That's part of the reason that the Canadian medical profession likes the Canadian system: Family doctors like it."

There was a brief doctors' strike in Ontario when the government banned extra billing. Until 1985, physicians could bill the government directly at the fee level set by negotiations between the government and the Medical Association, or they could bill the patient and the patient would collect the portion paid by the government. The patient would pay the difference between what the doctor billed and what the government paid. This practice is known in the United States as *balance billing* — when the doctor charges more than the insurance company or government program will pay.

The Canadian federal government outlawed this practice in the mid 1980s, using the power of the purse to enforce the change, and the provincial governments complied one by one. But there was significant opposition in Ontario, leading to a doctors' strike that inconvenienced many patients and resulted in what Detsky viewed as "a lot of political posturing."

"My perception is that the strike was really just a short blip in the general scheme of things," says Detsky. "It seems to me that physicians really are very much wedded to promoting the health system. Physicians work very much with the government to ensure that the system works. Only occasionally do the government and the doctors get into these scrapes.

"In my opinion, that Ontario strike was not what it appeared to be. There were many physicians who claimed to be on strike — yet, if you were to go examine their billings over the strike period, you would find that, although they may have been out carrying placards part of the time, they were still delivering care to their patients. It is very difficult for physicians to turn their back on their own patients and not deliver care they need. I think that strike was more of a media event than a real event."

Detsky acknowledges there are some drawbacks to the Canadian system, including "the well-known and much-publicized problem of waiting lines."

"It is clear that for some services in Canada, there are waiting lines that are uncomfortable for patients," he says. "These waits tend to be for sophisticated services such as diagnostic imaging techniques like magnetic resonance imagery and for cardiac surgery, lithotripsy, and, most recently, radiation therapy.

"It is important, though, to ask whether these waits are a reality or merely a perception. For cardiac surgery, waiting times seem to be longer in Canada than in the United States. Yet I recently received a phone call from an internist at the University of Vermont who expressed interest in learning about the Canadian triage system for cardiac surgery, which rates patients on a scale of urgency of need for treatment.

"I asked him, 'Why would you be interested in learning about this? Your patients have no waiting times.'

"'Oh, not so,' he said. 'Our waiting times are up to three months.'"

Detsky says there has been no fundamental study comparing waiting lines in the two countries.

Another disadvantage of the Canadian system is that it includes what Detsky terms "some fairly blunt supply constraints — that is, simple or arbitrary methods that limit the total size of hospital budgets." He says the effect of this "global budgeting" mechanism is to contain the growth of services delivered by institutions, thereby limiting supply and leaving little room for innovation in health care delivery systems. "For example, it's very difficult to introduce an HMO into the universal national health insurance system now in place in Canada," says Detsky.

A third problem area, he says, is "the question of how we measure quality of care."

"Media attention dictates the debate over resource shortages or perceived deficiencies in quality of care. This leads to political pressure and political action. The debate becomes too politicized.

"Future challenges to the Canadian health system won't be at the basic, fundamental level. The systems' structure is basically sound. It works. It works for government. It works for the public. And it works for providers, no matter what you might read in the newspapers."

The main challenge, he says, will be how to deal with new technologies that, despite their high cost, can have a positive impact on the health of individuals.

"I hope that, if any fundamental change does occur, it will be that we use a more rational, analytical process of decision making, instead of making decisions out in the media."

The question of how the Canadian system deals with cost controls is raised frequently: What goes on once a hospital or province has exceeded its health budget for the year and the year isn't over yet?

"There are periods when the provincial health costs do exceed the budget," says Detsky. "The provincial government then tries to balance the budget from one year to the next. There is no cutoff on provision of services, but there is a continual struggle to keep health care costs within the amounts budgeted.

"Portions of the budgeting process in all the provinces are open ended. The parts that are most open ended are those associated with fee-for-service reimbursement for professional fees, some drug costs, and some laboratory fees.

"Institutional costs are much more controlled. You have a certain number of dollars. That's all you get. Theoretically, a hospital might run out of money and stop treating patients, but in fact, that doesn't happen."

In those cases, the hospital might run a deficit and go to the government and try to get extra money, he says. It would then look for ways to reduce costs over the next year and get back in the black.

"If a hospital runs an operating deficit, the provincial government will become aware of it during the year and will sit down with the hospital administrators to see if they can come up with a plan to eliminate the deficit," says Detsky.

"There may be a good and sufficient reason the deficit cannot be eliminated. The community's population may have grown, or suddenly something new may have happened. Maybe AIDS has suddenly had a big impact. In such a case, the provincial government generally will come up with an additional subsidy. The hospital's global budget will be adjusted because there is a legitimate reason to do so."

Finally, Detsky says there has been a general recognition that too much care in Canada is provided in hospitals.

"At the same time, I think the government has been wise in being very cautious about moving services outside of institutions," he says. "If technology is moved outside the institutions, it becomes available in an environment that is less accountable, less controlled. You can't easily move high-tech services outside of institutions in Canada, because the provincial governments are very reluctant to fund these services. What the provincial governments have done is put pressure on hospitals to move services away from acute care beds but still keep those services in an organizational structure that is accountable and controlled."

Detsky says Canada has the opportunity to constrain the cost of new technology while still taking advantage of medical advances, because the government-run systems can balance need and cost.

"In the United States, a lot of new technology is untested," he says. "It gets out there, it becomes widespread, and then it's extremely difficult to contain. In Canada, it comes in very slowly and grows from the bottom up.

"I've recently seen statistics about the number of lithotripters (to dissolve kidney stones) in America. It's clear that the number of units that were brought on stream in America in 1988–89 vastly exceeds the demand for them. There was a back-log of cases, but these were treated in the 1986–87 period. And now there are a tremendous number of lithotripters out there with excess capacity. As a result, the benefit-risk ratio starts to drop. The same happens with all technologies.

"I tried to look for examples of treatments that are un-proven but nonetheless are widely disseminated," continues Detsky. "A carotid endarterectomy, an operation on the blood vessels in the neck, is a perfect example. This is a procedure aimed at reducing the incidence of strokes in people with athero-sclerosis in the vessels in their neck. It has never been proven to be of benefit. There's a good study showing that only a third of American patients who undergo the procedure, which is of unproven effectiveness, are even having it done for appropri-ate reasons.[1]

"This is the sort of problem you can prevent if you have the ability to contain new technologies."[2]

An Administrator's Perspective

While agreeing that the Canadian system offers workable meth-ods of restraining unnecessary growth of expensive new tech-nology, Vickery Stoughton's view from a hospital administra-tor's chair is that the restraints sometimes are too constricting and amount to a "wart" on the system.

"If the government errs, it errs on the side of being too slow," he says.

An example he cites is the small number of lithotripters in Canada relative to need — the flip side of Detsky's use of the same kidney stone–busting soundwave machines to underscore how the U.S. system can lead to unnecessary proliferation rela-tive to need.

Noting that there was one lithotripter to serve nine million people in Ontario in early 1992, Stoughton says: "We know litho-tripsy is cost effective, so this situation did not make any sense. This was a case where patients who needed to be treated and didn't want to wait for the one lithotripter would go somewhere else — to Buffalo or wherever. The government would pay for that travel, but as they started paying for it, they began to recognize that we really should add resources for this technology."

What happened next, however, underscored Stoughton's confidence that government does work with health care providers in an effort to measure cost against need and that "when we're all working together, generally we can figure out what the appropriate balance is." What happened next was that Ontario decided to add two more lithotripters.

Stoughton continues:

When we add those machines, we look at the incidence of need within the population base — in this case, the incidence of kidney stone disease. We conclude that, given the population base of nine million and the incidence of stone disease, we can justify between two and three of these machines in the province. Then the argument is about where to put them.

This is the process we generally go through. Health care costs continually rise — because of new technologies, inflation, and a host of other factors — and the province can't continually put more money into health care. So we've had to reallocate existing resources to pay for new technologies.

If you come into the Canadian health care system, you will find modern, efficient, comprehensive health care capabilities. But they aren't there because we've been constantly pumping new dollars into the system. The capabilities are there because internal resources have been reallocated to accommodate new technologies, within the financial constraints on the system. This has been happening in Ontario's institutions and in the rest of Canada's institutions over a period of ten to fifteen years.

The attempt to achieve an objective and reasoned allocation of resources, however, does not mean there are not political considerations in Canada, just as there are in the United States.

"As a result of the system's popularity, governments live

and die by the public perception of how the system is working,"
says Stoughton. "The result is that the health care system has
become highly politicized and is the subject of continuous media attention.

"Whenever there is a problem and the legislature is in session, the opposition party stands up in the legislature and asks
the minister of health to defend what's going on. There is always an effort on the part of opposition parties to create a public impression that the government is not staying on top of health
care affairs. If the opposition is successful in this, they're likely
to be successful in the next election."

One of the political realities, according to Stoughton, is
that hospitals in Canada are never shut down, no matter how
small or relatively inefficient when measured on a strict cost-
benefit ratio. "Of the 220 hospitals serving the nine million people
of Ontario," he says, "many are small ones — fewer than 100
beds — in rural areas that just do not close down because it would
be too politically sensitive to do so."

On the other hand, says Stoughton, "That's not to say
the system isn't coordinated." Most of these hospitals concentrate on providing the relatively low-tech care that is needed
in their communities and are not loaded with expensive high-
tech equipment that would sit idle most of the time.

"As a result, a lot of money is spent to transport patients
to centers offering expensive tertiary services such as cardiac
surgery, cancer treatment, transplants, and so forth," he says.
"If you live in a northern part of Ontario and you have a health
problem, you're given a check for $350 to get you to the center
that provides you with the diagnostic and treatment services you
need. If you can handle the ride, you can take a bus instead
of a commercial flight and pocket the difference in cost. If you're
sick enough, an airplane is sent to pick you up."

That's the way the Canadian system works. Sick Canadians get cared for under the government insurance program —
no matter where they are or what the medical problem may be.

"If a Canadian gets sick in Florida — really sick — the government payment branch does an assessment of whether to pay
for American treatment," said Stoughton. "Usually they conclude

that they shouldn't pay the American bills, and a plane is sent down to bring the sick person back to the Canadian system because it's cheaper to do so—including the cost of the plane."

Stoughton acknowledges that because Canadian hospitals' costs are controlled—and because technology and related high-level services are limited to hospitals—there sometimes are waiting lines for some procedures.

Still, he says the issue is a "red herring" in that it implies a fundamental problem with the system that simply doesn't exist. "Sometimes it might reflect a level of technology control that is temporarily inappropriate but that is self-correcting through public debate," argues Stoughton.

"Allocation of resources becomes a very open, very public, very political process. It takes place between the care providers, the physicians, the institutions, and the government. The public is able to judge the process openly."

He draws on his American background for comparison:

In my experience with cardiac surgery in Boston, the waiting times there were three to four months. The primary difference was that people in Boston had a choice of where to go for treatment. They could go to a center with perhaps less qualified, less well-known surgeons and get immediate cardiac care. But if they chose to go to Massachusetts General, the waiting times generally were three to four months. In the Canadian system, there is no opportunity to opt for a second-level facility. That is the primary difference between the two systems.

Because of the concentration of those services in so few centers in Canada, the quality of health care stands up to that of any system in the world. The people in these centers are experienced. The outcomes are good. The product these people produce serves the public extraordinarily well. Canada doesn't have centers doing too few cases. Canada doesn't have centers producing poor-quality care because of lack of experience.

In the province of Ontario, there are nine centers doing cardiac surgery. In the city of Toronto, which contains more than three million people, there are three cardiac surgery centers. Only one of the three is doing heart transplants.

Eventually, when population pressure develops to increase capacity for cardiac surgery, then new resources will be added. A fourth cardiac surgery center will be opened or a fourth new piece of equipment purchased, or whatever it takes to match the supply with the new demand.

Stoughton's position as an administrator dealing with recruitment of doctors in many different specialties gave him special insight into how the issue of comparative physician income in the United States and Canada plays out day to day in the real world.

He put it this way at a forum in Washington, D.C.:[3]

It has been suggested that the difference in physician fees between Canada and the United States might cause a brain drain of doctors from Canada to the United States. There's no question that the U.S. system has the capability of paying physicians more money, and that is a significant consideration. Canada tries to recruit people all the time from the United States for medical and management leadership positions, so Canadians have become familiar with American salary levels.

If you take a general surgeon in Canada making $200,000 or a thoracic surgeon in Canada making $240,000 and compare that with an American surgeon making $400,000 or $500,000, there is a significant difference.

The other part of the equation is that when you practice medicine in the United States, you've got unbelievable hassles. You're paying for medical malpractice insurance at a much higher rate than in Canada. And there are overhead costs that are significantly higher than overheads in Canada.

Canadian doctors who have gone to the United States say U.S. doctors do not enjoy the same kind of freedom of practice in America as they did in Canada. These Canadian physicians have come away with an unfavorable opinion of the American system, even though it is richer economically than the Canadian system.

Overall, the Canadian fee schedules run about 20 to 30 percent lower than in the United States, depending on which area of the country you're comparing with. One might think this would be a problem in terms of losing Canadian doctors to America. But we have looked at this question very closely at the University of Toronto and at The Toronto Hospital: Canada just does not lose many doctors to the United States.

Stoughton says hospitals in Canada employ many fewer full-time employees on average than hospitals in the United States, except at teaching hospitals, where the ratio of between 4 and 4.5 full-time positions per bed is about the same as for U.S. teaching hospitals.

Community hospitals, in particular, have reduced the number of full-time positions per bed, because the concentration of high technology in a relatively few high-volume institutions enables the smaller institutions to care for their relatively less sick patient population with relatively less staff.

But Stoughton contends that because the higher-end technology is confined to hospitals in Canada — as opposed to standalone diagnostic and specialized treatment facilities — there is an overuse of institutional care in Canada compared to the United States.

"For example, the number of patient days per 1,000 population in Canada is in the neighborhood of 1,300, compared to around 1,000 in the United States," he says.

A Business Executive's Perspective

Most Canadian autoworkers are based in the province of Ontario, with a good number in Quebec as well. Some are scattered throughout the rest of the provinces, mostly in regional sales offices and parts depots. This pattern holds true for all the Big Three automakers: Chrysler, Ford, and General Motors.

It is a situation not unlike what William Fisher was familiar with as a Chrysler executive in the United States, where employees tended to be concentrated in the Midwest but also were spread among other regions.

In each Canadian province, autoworkers are covered by the provincial health insurance plan, just like everyone else. The provincial plans differ, but Fisher explains that the auto industry in Canada takes the Ontario provincial insurance program as a standard.

"If in any particular province the public health insurance does not provide coverage up to the Ontario standard, the auto companies will provide private insurance to make up the difference," he says. "In this way, autoworkers throughout Canada enjoy a standard level of health insurance coverage from coast to coast."

Although the differences among the provinces' plans are relatively minor, a fair amount of work is involved in coming up with a standard coverage for all of a company's employees across the country. A private insurance carrier is used to smooth out the differences.

"It would be difficult for us to transfer our employees from one province to another if such a transfer might move an employee from a situation where there was extensive health coverage to one where the coverage was not as good," says Fisher. "For example, you can't expect an employee to accept a transfer from Ontario to some other province if this would mean giving up the free annual eye examination offered under Ontario's plan."

In addition, the automakers provide private insurance that covers some services not included under the provincial plans — semiprivate hospital accommodations, for example, rather than the ward accommodation that is the basic benefit under the Ontario government insurance plan.

Other add-on examples include a prescription drug plan, a dental plan, a vision plan that covers contact lenses and eyeglass frames, and a hearing aid plan.

The automakers also provide private insurance to cover some of the copayments required for nursing home care and

for certain prosthetic devices and durable medical equipment
such as walkers and wheelchairs that may not be covered by
the government plan.

"The private insurance provided by the auto industry also
includes supplementary coverage for out-of-province surgical
and medical expenses," continues Fisher. "For example, if I were
injured in Washington, D.C., I would have coverage, under
the industry's private insurance, for the 'reasonable and custo-
mary' expense of medical care in Washington, as measured against
what the Ontario public insurance program would provide."

All of the auto plans are provided by a private insurance
carrier, Green Shield Prepaid Services Inc., based in Toronto.
The firm started in the city of Windsor, Ontario, and grew from
there. It now writes insurance policies across the country and
is used extensively by all the auto companies.

Employees at Ford, Chrysler, and General Motors have
identical coverage paid by the companies. Other industries in
Canada provide similar comprehensive private insurance, although not always as extensive as the automobile industry. But
many of the larger ones — such as the steel or pulp and paper
industries — pay for vision and dental care.

Still, the comprehensive private insurance programs do
not cover nearly all of the workers in Canada.

"I would estimate that about 25 percent of Canadians have
extra private insurance in addition to their provincial public
health insurance," says Fisher.

The autoworkers' coverage is fully paid for by the auto
companies. The insurance covers the employee and his or her
eligible dependents while the worker is actively employed by
the company and for several months after active employment
in the event of layoff or disability leave. It also covers retired
employees and their eligible dependents.

With the government insurance program as a foundation,
Fisher is firm in his belief that the Canadian system works for
management and employees as well:

I think it is safe to say that Canadian autoworkers are very
comfortable and well satisfied with their comprehensive

health care coverage. They and their families are well protected, and they are covered not only during their working career but also after retirement.

Health care complaints from employees and retirees in the Canadian auto industry are few and far between. In my many years of working in the auto industry in the personnel and human resources area, we had very few complaints, from either union or nonunion employees, with respect to their health care coverage. The coverage is something that has been there for many years. It's taken for granted that autoworkers will receive this benefit, and it's much appreciated by them.

I think the Canadian workers I've worked with over the years are a healthier group than the U.S. workers I've worked with. One of the reasons is that many of the Canadians take advantage of a provision in the provincial health plans that covers annual physical examinations.

One of the basic differences between the two systems over the years has been that home and office visits are covered in Canada. In the United States, these home and office visits are not provided. I think a result is that, if employees have to pay for such visits, they may not bother to see the doctor at all. And they might end up with serious illnesses that could have been avoided.

By making life and health better for workers, the setup in Canada makes life easier for management as well, Fisher explains.

"Even though health care coverage is one of our principal benefits, it has not been a major issue in recent negotiations," says Fisher. "It was not a major issue in talks with the Canadian Auto Workers Union in 1987, 1985, or 1982. Other matters, such as pension indexation and general wage increases, have been the major issues. In the recent past, very little attention has been paid to health care in the course of labor negotiations.

"Most of the significant changes in the health care coverage were negotiated in the 1960s and the early 1970s. In the negotiations, for example, health care demands of the unions were few in number and modest in cost."

By contrast, Fisher is well aware of what his management counterparts in the United States have been going through in labor negotiations that focus with increasing ferocity on health benefit issues.

He was directly involved with labor negotiations with Chrysler U.S. workers for many years before 1977 and after 1977 was involved with negotiations for Chrysler Canada.

"In the United States, health care has been a principal issue on the table in each round of negotiations in the last ten years," he says. "I know it has been discussed extensively. The companies would like to change the coverage offered, moving toward systems of copayment and arrangements that would reduce the cost and share the cost among the employers and the employees.

"Health care has been a much bigger issue in the United States than in Canada in recent years. Certainly labor negotiations over health benefits are more subject to impasse in the United States. In Canada, there hasn't been as much pressure to switch from the current system of benefits, because health care costs there haven't been nearly as high."

Fisher elaborates:

From about 1967 until the CAW pulled out of the UAW in 1985, Chrysler had an international labor agreement. We negotiated all wages and benefits, including health care, at one time. The agreement covered both Canadian and U.S. employees. Whatever health care changes were adopted in the United States were either adopted in Canada, or adapted to the Canadian situation and then adopted. Since 1985, we've had to negotiate a separate agreement for Canada.

Canadian health care costs are significantly higher than those in Japan, Korea, and West Germany. Canadian firms compete directly with manufacturers in these countries. Our production costs must be carefully monitored, and cost controls must be implemented wherever possible for Canadian automakers to continue to be competitive in the world marketplace.

The industry is concerned about the recent trend of coverage cost increases. Health care is our third most expensive benefit, after pension plans and vacation pay. Inflation in the cost of health benefits has ranged from 10 to 20 percent yearly since 1984; the figure varies for the different benefits. The two health care benefits where cost increases are the most worrisome are the prescription drug and dental plans.

The Canadian Auto Workers Union has taken a responsible position with respect to health care cost control. The labor agreement provides for a joint labor-management committee to make sure the money spent on premiums delivers the optimum benefits. In addition, this committee also reviews the annual cost-containment reports issued by the insurance carriers. The committee may investigate potential cost-saving measures and, on mutual agreement, enact them.

In 1987, the Canadian Auto Workers' settlement included negotiated changes in health coverage that resulted in some health cost reductions, primarily in some of the supplementary benefits.

Generally speaking, the auto industry employers feel that all components of the comprehensive plan are very well administered. This applies to the parts administered by the private insurance carrier as well as to the parts administered by the provinces.

For all of Fisher's enthusiasm for the Canadian health care system from a hard-eyed business perspective, he is equally impressed on other grounds.

He notes with the relish of a busy executive that he hasn't had to deal with a doctor bill or hassle with an insurance company on a personal level for years and, even more personally, has had firsthand exposure to the inherent convenience, effectiveness, and humaneness of the whole system.

"Last week my eighty-nine-year old father had a lens transplant in Windsor, Ontario," Fisher recounted during a recent talk to a U.S. audience. "This was done in a hospital by an ophthalmologist who specializes in surgical work. He went into the hospital at 9:00 in the morning, and he was home eating his lunch at 12:30.

"I had to take my father to the doctor the next day for a follow-up exam in the doctor's office at no cost to my father. He was examined, and everything was fine, and he said, 'You know, it's nice to have good, capable doctors taking care of the old folks.'

"And the doctor said to him, 'It's nice to have good, old patients like you, Mr. Fisher.'"

CHAPTER 4

Voices from the Polls:
Consensus and Satisfaction
from Canadian Patients and Taxpayers

Ian McKinnon

The Canadian health care system ranks higher in popularity than any other major social system in Canada—higher than the very popular education system or a variety of other analogous services.

In one survey, Canadians were shown the statement: "One of the things that makes Canada the best country in the world in which to live is the quality and availability of our health care system." Fully 90 percent of the respondents agreed with the assertion.[1]

Comparisons of surveys show dramatic differences in satisfaction with the health care systems of Canada and the United States. Harris polls in 1988 asked Canadians and Americans whether "on the whole the health care system works pretty well and only minor changes are necessary to make it better," "there are some good things in our health care system but fundamental changes are needed to make it work better," or "our health care system has so much wrong with it that we need to completely rebuild it." A majority of Canadians (56 percent) said their system works pretty well, but only 10 percent of the Americans held that view.[2]

One of the things that really struck me while going over our data was the fact that when American survey researchers ask about health care systems, they include questions about issues we do not ask about in Canada. Americans ask about personal feelings of risk to the family if there is a serious illness. I looked through our data banks from the 100 to 200 surveys Decima has done for ten years. We've never asked about fears of medical expenses, simply because this concern is not one of the operating assumptions Canadians make about their health care system.

Our basic measure of satisfaction is assessment of quality. In one set of surveys of Canadians, we asked each respondent to assess the quality of the health care available in his or her province. The results show that there has been very little change in response to this question over time. The data run from 1983 through 1987. Twenty-nine percent said the quality of care was excellent, 48 percent said good, 17 percent said only fair, and 6 percent said poor.[3]

We checked whether people during this same time period felt that the health care system, even if it was a good one, was deteriorating or improving. We found that the largest percentage of people — 47 percent in our most recent survey — said there has been no change recently in the quality of health care in their community. More people say it has improved than it has deteriorated, by a 35 to 18 percent margin.[4]

I have analogous American data that indicate that, if we ask Americans whether their system is improving or deteriorating, 27 percent say it has improved, 20 percent say it has deteriorated, and 49 percent say there has been no change.[5]

So, even on the margins, not only are Canadians significantly more satisfied with the quality of their health care system than are Americans with their system, but Canadians also are more likely to say that the Canadian system is, in fact, improving.

Canadians recognize many of the same challenges that face the United States. Even if Canada is spending a significantly lower proportion of its gross national product (GNP) on health care, Canadians nonetheless say their system's health care costs are increasing. In fact, 66 percent of Canadians say that health care costs are rising more rapidly than the general cost of living.[6] They are aware of the problem because it is such a high-profile political issue, not because they are themselves having to pay for it. They are aware of it because they are seeing the issue raised in the legislatures.

The kinds of solutions to cost problems offered by Canadians are very similar to those suggested in the United States. There is widespread support across Canada for preventive medicine and the promotion of healthier life-styles. Two-thirds of our Canadian respondents agreed with the statement, "The government wouldn't spend so much on health care if they spent more time and money promoting healthier life-styles."[7]

So, Canadians give responses very similar to those of Americans on public policy questions, if not to questions about other more personal questions of cost containment.

One of the striking things about the Canadian system is that Canadians don't perceive there to be a very strong link between the amount a person uses the system and that person's level of health knowledge. Once we asked whether people felt that providing citizens with health education or a grounding in health knowledge — something that isn't done now — would reduce abuse of the system. A majority, but only a pretty bare majority of 56 percent said this would help.[8]

What is interesting in this and related questions is that most Canadians believe free and unlimited access to the health care system does not contribute to rising health costs in any significant way.

Let me draw a comparison between the Canadian picture and American data, again from the Cambridge Reports group. They asked, at the end of 1987, "Do you think all Americans should have access to the same quality of health care, regardless of their ability or not to pay for it?" Eighty-five percent agreed.[9]

They also asked, "Do you think it should be up to the government to provide good health care for all Americans, whether or not they can afford it?" This question specifically proposed health care as a government responsibility. Seventy-one percent agreed; 16 percent disagreed.

To me, these answers are relatively compelling evidence that, despite differences in policy, we are not dealing with two dramatically different cultures. We do not find something peculiar and unique about the country north of the 49th parallel that causes its citizens to embrace a value system that is dramatically different from the American system.

Over and over again, when we do comparative studies, we find that the two countries' beliefs on many issues aren't that different. What *is* different is the experience that Canadians have had over the last twenty-five to thirty years with a radically different health care system—experience that has led to very, very high levels of approval of that system.

Decima Research has done a lot of polling on both sides of the border. I think it is fundamentally a myth that Americans view their government dramatically differently than Canadians view their government, and that Americans trust their government less than Canadians do theirs.

There are indications that on certain issues where Canadians have been habituated to government involvement, they may more readily countenance government involvement in areas Americans would find unusual. But when it comes to fundamental trust in government generally, and the degree to which government is perceived to be serving the needs of the public over the desires and political goals of the selfish few, there isn't much difference between the two countries.

Canadians are just as hostile to their governments as are Americans. In fact, Canada has a higher rate of government turnover than America has. Canada defeats its governments more frequently. But Canadians trust government as an agency.

The doctors' strike in Ontario in 1986 over the question of balance billing provided an opportunity to understand Canadian attitudes toward key aspects of the system. Decima Research was in the field doing public policy research during the strike period. Two very interesting things happened.

One is that the strike brought to the fore an issue that Canadians don't like to deal with: the notion that access or your place in the queue is in some way dependent on having the finances to pay for things like balance billing. As this issue gained prominence and salience during the strike—*work action* would really be a better term for it than *strike*—the numbers showed people becoming incredibly opposed to the idea. It's not that waiting in line is popular. Rather, the idea of being able to jump the line depending on one's financial status is very unpopular.

The other very interesting consequence of the strike was that it made the Ontario medical profession realize the depth of solid, fundamental support by the public for the basic principles of the Canadian medical system. I watched and dealt with people on both sides of the issue during that period, and this was very interesting. Until there was this moment of truth, doctors could say, "Well, people accept balance billing. They want the access it buys, and so they're really on our side." It was an eye-opening experience for many in the medical profession.

I also think the strike was an anomaly. It's going to happen very, very rarely. And I think it reaffirmed the fundamentals of the system.

There are some differences between the American and Canadian systems.

The first is the level of satisfaction with the system. Canadians all across the country show a higher level of satisfaction with their health care than Americans show with their system.

The second major difference is what is or is not on the health care agenda. That's perhaps the most interesting question. It's rather like Sherlock Holmes saying that what's important is that the dog didn't bark. In this case, what's important is the lack of fear at the household level about the economic consequences of illness. This is simply not an issue in Canada. In focus groups in Canada, I have raised the question of worries about health care expenses. To put it bluntly, it takes a considerable length of time for a typical Canadian to understand the issue of fear of economic consequences of illness. Canadians find it difficult to believe that as affluent a country as the United States could allow that kind of problem to occur. They simply don't understand it.

Canadians view two main factors as the basis of their health system. One is their belief that everyone should have full access to the system. Now, Canadians realize that if you live in downtown Toronto you may have a somewhat different level of access to health care than if you live somewhere in northern Manitoba. Canadians aren't utterly impractical about access. Rather, we feel that access to health care should not be a function of personal economic wealth or position.

The second fundamental point contributing to the high approval ratings of the Canadian system is that it offers choice. People have choice over the physicians they see. They have choice over the hospitals they visit.

These two factors, choice and access, are the twin attributes that underpin Canadians' favorable views of their health care system.

One important difference between the Canadian and American systems has to do with who negotiates decisions. The distinction here is between the American system of negotiation between doctors and insurers, and the Canadian system of negotiation between doctors and the government. And the Canadian version is one of the main reasons Canadians have so much confidence in their system. Fundamentally, Canadians trust both their doctors and their government. These two groups are perceived to act in Canadians' best interests.

This perception contrasts sharply with some perceptions in the United States. There, people do tend to trust doctors, but Americans have no specific reason to trust the other players, the insurance companies. The problem is the whole issue of whether Americans have confidence in the system and in the people who design the system's rationing mechanisms.

Similar problems confront both the Canadian and American health care systems. Cost containment is a problem in both countries. Questions surrounding technological change and the introduction and dissemination of technology are issues in Canada and America alike.

Because the government runs the Canadian health care system, health care problems here are highly visible and are political problems. Consequently, these problems immediately become high-profile issues for the press and for opposition parties.

Something that happened in the 1988 Canadian election illustrates how fundamental Canadians' views about their health care system are.

The primary issue in that election was the free trade agreement with the United States. Opponents said throughout the campaign that one of the big problems with the agreement was that it might put the Canadian health care system at risk. While critics of the agreement also argued that it would undermine Canadian culture and identity, it was only the assertion that the health care system would be endangered that really affected people.

Decima was doing political survey research throughout that campaign and found the ads about the threat to the Canadian health care system were very successful. The ads forced the government to rethink its election campaign and change strategy to provide the most sweeping assertions possible that a free trade agreement with the United States would not in any way jeopardize the Canadian health care system. That is a measure of how important this system is to Canadians. And it is a measure of the degree to which the issue is seen to have become part of Canada's fundamental social fabric.

There hasn't been a serious debate about anything verging on the fundamentals of the health care system in twenty years. It's inviolable across the political spectrum, from the mildly socialist New Democrats on the one end, through the Liberals and Progressive Conservatives, all the way to the right-wing Social Credit Party on the other side. The health care system is accepted broadly.

I think future health care questions will be relatively hard fought and intense on the political level. But these questions will concern the margins of the health care system, not its fundamentals. The kinds of issues that Canada faces now are questions about moving from institutionalized care toward community-based care, about wellness programs, and about how health programs can be integrated with other social programs.

I do not foresee any argument arising in Canada in the near future about any of the basics of the health care system. The consensus is too wide. There is agreement that the system works well, and satisfaction levels are simply too high to permit serious challenges.

CHAPTER 5

The Political Perspective:
Planning and Implementing the Canadian System

The Honorable Allan E. Blakeney

I want to issue a disclaimer at the outset: I am not a doctor, and I am not an expert on medical care. I'm a lawyer and a politician. In some respects, we're like journalists. We are experts in everything or nothing, depending on whether you believe us or you believe our victims. I have some knowledge of medical care gained while participating in government and wrestling with some of the problems of setting up an appropriate medical care insurance program. But I have no expertise in the medical services delivered to patients.

Canada's health insurance program has roots that go back as far as the days of pioneer settlement in the Canadian prairies. Many communities developed plans where the local government would hire doctors and pay all or part of the doctors' salaries. These physicians were called *municipal doctors*. These local plans continued in rudimentary form right up until World War II. Following World War II, there was considerable expansion of nonprofit insurance plans for hospital care and other medical care. These were of the Blue Cross/Blue Shield variety and were sponsored by hospitals and medical associations.

Saskatchewan is a Western province of about a million people. Its topography is something like that of western Minnesota, or North Dakota, or eastern Montana. In 1947, it was largely agricultural. In that year, the provincial government established a plan to provide insurance for hospital care. Each person or family paid an annual premium and was entitled to have any basic hospital bills paid. The plan was universal: everybody was covered, and everybody paid the premium. So, in effect, the premium was a kind of tax.

The government negotiated rates of payment with the hospitals. At that time, as is true today, almost all hospitals in Saskatchewan were owned and operated by either municipal governments or religious organizations. Under the plan, hospitals were paid for their services out of the funds collected through premiums. If the premiums taken in were insufficient to cover costs, any shortfalls were made up out of general provincial revenues.

At the same time that the Saskatchewan hospital insurance plan was launched, a program was started jointly by the federal and Saskatchewan governments to pay the capital costs of constructing new hospitals.

The plans for renewing hospital facilities and for insuring hospital services went forward simultaneously, and both were well received by the public and the hospitals alike. There were the inevitable administrative hassles, but there was no opposition to the plan in principle.

By 1957, the idea of hospital care insurance had spread to other provinces. The federal government became interested, and in 1958 it launched a proposal to pay half the costs of hospital insurance in any provinces where these costs were insured by a comprehensive provincial plan. And so, shortly thereafter, comprehensive hospital plans were in operation in all ten Canadian provinces.

A few years later, a similar thing happened with medical care insurance. We started a program in Saskatchewan and it soon was adapted for all of Canada by the federal government.

Before we get into the hard-core politics, let me try to give you a little feel for how this all evolved in Saskatchewan.

The frontier, pioneering nature of our society required that people work together to survive. It is a very, very harsh climate. In the early days of settlement, people either worked together or they perished — sometimes literally. They organized small school districts in which people got together and built the schoolhouse with their own labor. They paid their taxes and they went out and found the schoolteacher.

If you go into rural Saskatchewan today, almost every community hall would be a result of that kind of cooperation. That's how they got things done as late as the 1970s.

Every little town has its ice rink. It's a center of activity where people gather to pass time during the long winters.

I'll give you one example of how a little town of about 1,000 people got its rink. These people simply didn't have the money to have it built, so they said among themselves: "Here it is. You know what rinks are made of. They are made of cement, and we'll get some cement. And they're made of wood. There are plenty of trees here, so let's go to see the government and get ourselves a permit to cut some government-owned trees."

So they cut and hauled logs out of the forest with their farm tractors and set up a little sawmill. They let the lumber dry for a year. And then they built their rink. I could give you a number of similar stories. All of this is done informally. There is no committee. But it gets done. These are not 1913 stories, these are 1975 stories and this is still going on.

So that tradition of cooperation is deeply rooted in rural Canada.

I have mentioned municipal doctors. Later, this same tradition was at work when the municipalities got together and organized larger districts and built district hospitals. There are dozens of them now. They're called *Union* hospitals. "Plainsview Union Hospital," for example, would be the result of towns X, Y, and Z getting together to build a hospital.

There was a great wave of that kind of building immediately after World War II, in the 1940s and 1950s. This all preceded the present structure of provincewide hospital and physician insurance.

This was a continuation of a tradition of people getting together to deal with the costs of catastrophic illness. In the 1920s, the rural municipalities bonded together to provide care without cost to the patient for what was then the scourge, tuberculosis. Later the province provided care for the mentally ill.

Again there was no payment at the time the service was delivered, although there were rights to claim against the estate of a deceased mental patient.

Free cancer treatment was offered in 1945. The treatment was organized by the medical profession, who believed that there was a lot of less-than-top-grade professional surgery going on for cancer. They thought that the government should not pay for any services until the patients had first gone through a cancer clinic at Regina or Saskatoon, our largest cities, and were evaluated by competent people.

That is basically how it operates to this day, although it has loosened up somewhat. But certainly up until 1960, virtually every surgical procedure for cancer was done in a cancer clinic by a person who was skilled in cancer surgery.

I don't want to dwell on it too much, but it is important to understand that these traditions of cooperation — for purely pragmatic reasons — were well entrenched in rural Canada before the politicians got into the health care business at the provincial and national levels.

Now, on to the politics.

It started with a confluence of circumstances and personalities. A lot of what we have in Canada now in the way of health care goes back to Tommy Douglas, who was elected premier of Saskatchewan in 1944 and who was passionately interested in health. He was so involved that he kept the health portfolio himself for the first four years or so as premier. That might be a little like a U.S. governor keeping day-to-day operating control over a state health department.

Tommy Douglas had all sorts of health problems when he was a boy. He had a problem with his leg that could have left him crippled. His father was a skilled printer in Winnipeg. But in the 1920s, when Tommy was a teenager, printers just could not afford high-grade surgical treatment. Nonetheless Tommy got the care he needed because some doctor who was interested in the case agreed to take care of him for a fee his father could afford. Because of the good treatment given him, Tommy subsequently became an amateur boxer and, among other things, a stage performer and a brilliant elocutionist.

He regarded the recovery that enabled him to do these

things as something that had come to him by pure accident,
sheer luck. I suppose he would say it was by divine grace, and
he was going to see that he spread around the divine grace as
much as he could. He had that passion when he became premier, and he was a very, very strong-willed man, very able and
bright. Charismatic. Stubborn.

There was a degree of opposition when the provincewide
hospital plan was introduced in 1947. But it was not substantial. The reasons were clear. The hospitals were operated by
the same people who previously operated them, local boards.
The role of the province was to pay the bills, as a nongovern-
ment insurer would do.

At any rate, the Saskatchewan hospital insurance plan
was soon well in place. In 1958, the federal government produced
national hospital insurance and began to pay half the tab, with
the provinces paying the other half. This was a bonanza for
Saskatchewan.

By 1959, the talk in Saskatchewan had turned to a medical care plan to pay doctor bills, and the 1960 election was fought
on that issue. I campaigned on this issue. Everyone campaigned
on this issue.

It was my first election and I was running for a multimem-
ber seat. I had an arrangement with my running mate where
she would talk about welfare and housing and I would talk about
workers' compensation and jobs. We decided we would both
talk about medical care, because it might turn out to be a big
issue. As it turned out, medical care was all we could talk about.
It became the only issue. That's all the public was talking about,
all anybody was talking about.

Our party wanted to run on our record and on rural roads
and getting electrical power to the last batch of farms. These
had always been powerful issues. We thought: "Well, people
will still be interested in roads. When is the time people in rural
Saskatchewan are not going to be interested in roads? That day
is not going to dawn."

We thought the health plan would be one of the four or
five major issues, but it rapidly became *the* issue. I think one
reason is that the medical profession fought so hard against it.

If our party spent "X" dollars on the campaign, the doctors spent "X plus." I don't know the exact figures, but they clearly spent more than we did — and more than our opposition party did. I think the doctors changed the nature of the campaign with their advertising campaign. There is no question that the health plan would have been an issue, but it quickly became the number one issue because doctors were so vehemently and publicly opposed to it. Their theme was: "Political Medicine is Bad Medicine."

As it worked out, I don't think anyone could question the fact that the 1960 election in Saskatchewan was one in which the absolutely overarching issue was the introduction of a medical care plan. The doctors were on one side and the Co-operative Commonwealth Federation, or CCF, as we were known then, was on the other side. The other political parties were a bit ambivalent.

(Our party, the CCF, later became the NDP, the New Democratic Party.)

I do not recall the doctors flatly saying "Don't vote CCF," but they made it absolutely, blindingly clear with their television ads that voting against us was what they wanted the people to do.

Some of our opponents attacked us as proponents of "socialized medicine." Tommy Douglas would say: "Well, I don't know whether it is socialized medicine or not. I'm just talking about making sure that the doctor bill gets paid if your child gets sick." He was a pretty pragmatic soul, and he got the debate off the high ideological plane.

So we won that election in what amounted to a referendum on the health care plan we supported. But there was no question that real apprehension remained on the part of the public because the campaign had been very, very vigorous. I can remember some of the speeches by the doctors. They were sent out in a kit to all the doctors in the province. (We got copies because we had some doctors who were quite sympathetic to us.)

Those speeches had lines in them like: "What will happen when the medical care plan comes in? All the local doctors will leave. British doctors will not practice under this plan; they know all about state medicine. You will be left with nothing but the garbage of the art." Clearly that was meant to characterize doctors from places other than Britain. And that was incredible, because less than half the people in Saskatchewan are of English or French origin. A very large number are from other countries of Europe. So I went around to the Romanian Hall or the Hungarian Hall making sure they knew what the doctors were saying.

But the organized medical profession was successful in creating in the public mind the idea that the doctors would not stay once we put the plan into practice. (The public body created to oppose the medical care plan during the crisis months of April, May, and June of 1961 was called "Keep Our Doctors" or "K.O.D." for short.) Even though we felt that most of the doctors would stay, as in fact they did, the medical people played it shrewdly. At one point during the Medicare dispute, they put up a big "For Sale" sign in front of a clinic in Saskatoon. It wasn't that there was anyone to buy the building, but the sign made their point. There was a lot of that kind of hype.

There coalesced a group of people eager for political office who thought they could organize public support against the medical plan — not the idea of a medical plan, mind you, but the particular plan that we put in place. The interesting thing is that by the time they got into power in 1964, they did not dare try to dislodge the medical care plan, which was working quite well by that time and was well received by the public.

But the political discontent with us had been sown earlier. This stemmed from a well-known phenomenon among politicians: the public does not like the process of change. People like the results of change, but they do not like the process. You are likely to have a tough year for any major new program, and perhaps we underestimated how tough it would be with regard to our medical care program. We did not think anyone could mount a successful campaign against medical care, given the history of Saskatchewan. But it was done. It would not last long, but it was done for a short time. I could not have won if I had been up for reelection in 1962. In 1960 I was fine, and by 1964 I was fine. But not in 1962.

There were no provincial elections that year, but Douglas

was a candidate for the federal House of Commons for a Regina seat. This was during the time the medical care crisis was in full swing, during the run-up to the doctor's strike. Douglas was defeated, and the major reason was public apprehension about medical care. I was busy campaigning with Tommy, and there was no doubt what the problem was. If you had held a referendum on the plan during the period between the time the bill was passed and the time the plan was up and running, you would have lost it.

Douglas soon was to play a pivotal role in setting in motion the events that led to the national health plan we have now. But the New Democrats did very badly in that national election, and there is no question that, in Saskatchewan, the medical plan had a lot to do with our losses. In that sense, the doctors carried the day during that one period of a few months leading up to the 1962 elections.

The act setting up the plan was passed in the fall of 1961, and by the following April, the doctors really began to get themselves cranked up. They had a mass meeting in May and said they would not practice under the plan. They all put up signs in their offices saying they would close when the plan was implemented July 1. By mid-June they were telling people they were not booking any surgery, because after July 1 the hospitals would not be operating.

All this, of course, was done with the greatest sympathy for their patients. The doctors would tell them how sorry they were the government was making them stop treating their patients and that perhaps they could arrange for them to leave Saskatchewan and go to Winnipeg in Manitoba or Calgary in Alberta for treatment. All this kind of stuff was pouring out over a period of six weeks or two months. They were careful to say they would run emergency services "in case your life is threatened, but until this is sorted out we will not practicing under the government plan. We probably won't charge anything." It went on and on and on. You could not go to a doctor's office without being lobbied.

The plan went into effect July 1, as we promised, and the doctors went on strike, as they promised.

But public support was leaning in favor of the plan and the reaction by our government to the striking doctors was: "Okay, it's too bad, but if you're going, you're going. We can bring in doctors, and the licensed English doctors here will share the load for the time being until we get the new doctors."

By and large, we were our own public relations consultants. We had advertising agencies but, at that time, they simply placed the ads and assisted in drafting the ads. They were not, in any sense, public relations consultants as that term is now understood.

I don't know whether the Saskatchewan College of Physicians and Surgeons had public relations consultants or not. I have always assumed they did. There were some people from the Canadian Medical Association around from time to time during the prestrike and strike periods, but I am just not aware of the extent to which they used outside public relations people.

There was a little bit of hardball for about seventeen days, and then the "emergency services" got better and better. It seems the striking doctors were considering more and more ailments to be "emergencies."

No politician ever says "never," but we felt at this point that we were going to play it until the end. We knew it would be tough, but it was July and people don't get sick much in July. They go on holidays. As a matter of fact, a lot of the doctors went on holiday, too. They said: "Okay, we'll wait two or three weeks and see how things are going. We don't mind being out of our offices a few weeks in July. Who would? This thing has to settle."

We knew that a fair number of the doctors were very uncertain about their position. They wanted to go along with the College of Physicians and Surgeons, the medical organization, and not rock the boat. They were apprehensive about the plan on two levels, one of which was totally unfounded and one of which was not totally unfounded.

They said they were worried that the government would interfere, in a major way, with the way they practiced — tell them to treat measles on Mondays and do appendectomies on Thursdays, or whatever. They did not believe the "measles on Monday" silliness for a minute, but a number of them did fear that there would be enough regulation to, say, limit the number of appendectomies they could perform. This was ill-founded, but I think a number of them really did believe there would be unacceptable limits on what they could do. They just had no experience with these things at all.

Their viewpoint was that they had been "good doctors" in the sense that they had been faithful doctors, not making vast incomes or gouging their patients. At least by their perceptions, they had not been overservicing patients because there were lots of patients. They saw themselves as a socially responsible lot set upon by these politicians who wanted to curry votes by promising all sorts of things.

That was their thinking, and they did not have the slightest idea how the government operates.

I remember speaking with them and they would say, "But who is making the decisions?" I would answer, "Well, the cabinet decides. People sit down, they discuss it, and some consensus is arrived at." They just did not believe that. They thought some Machiavellian hand was guiding everything. I don't know exactly what they thought, but it was strange. These were rational, intelligent human beings, but they were in such a state of alarm and so unfamiliar with how any government works that it was difficult to even engage them rationally.

The other thing they felt, with considerable justification, was that this ultimately was going to affect their incomes because governments would somehow want to control costs. That was not well founded in the sense that it was going to happen tomorrow or next year, but over the long haul, I think there is no doubt that public insurance schemes affect the ability of doctors to set fees one way or another.

They made the assumption that if the insurance scheme were not there, they would have an untrammeled right to set fees. But they overlooked the fact that they did not have an untrammeled right to *collect* them because there are very clear limitations to what you can collect from the public.

Doctors who had practiced in Saskatchewan for some time—particularly those who had memories of Saskatchewan in the 1930s, many of whom had problems in collecting 60 or 70 cents on the dollar over the years — were not overly worried about arguing with the government over their fees. They could see the possibility of being better off on balance because at least the government could guarantee payment.

But many of the specialists and others were very concerned on that score. The medical hierarchy is heavily influenced by specialists, who do have a pretty good ability to set and collect fees because we are relatively short of specialists. They were the leaders of the profession then and still are almost everywhere.

The leaders in Saskatchewan had a good number of discussions with the Canadian Medical Association, which, I think, urged them to take a stand against medical care insurance to the extent they could and offered them lots of help. We suspect, but cannot absolutely establish, that the American Medical Association was working with the Canadian Medical Association to assist them in taking a stand.

At any rate, the rank-and-file doctors were willing to go along with their organization, and so they closed their offices.

That started the dynamic of huge media attention. Normally, ten reporters at a news conference in Regina is a mob, and during this period we were having two-a-day news conferences with sixty or seventy there from Los Angeles and Washington and London and all over. A doctors' strike was a much rarer commodity then than it is now.

We began to bring in doctors from the United Kingdom, and the striking doctors probably knew we also had arrangements with a couple of groups in the United States to bring in doctors if we needed them — from a steelworkers' medical plan in Pittsburgh and from a medical group in Detroit. We could have brought in teams of specialists if we had had to, as well as people to cover emergency services if the doctors pulled those.

I have never seen anything in my political life like the level of social controversy during that time.

Everybody had an opinion: people who had never been bothered with politics before or since. I had more irate and angry telephone calls at night than ever before or since. Police kept an eye on the home of Premier Lloyd and that sort of thing. This kind of security may not seem strange now, but it was then.

A charismatic Catholic priest who was violently opposed to the medical care plan gave a speech early on in the strike in which he more or less said, "If the government does not withdraw this bill and withdraw it now, there will be blood running in the streets and God help us if it does not." Now this is fairly vigorous language for a Catholic priest to say God help us if blood doesn't run in the street.

Actually, we were a little pleased with that, because many of the opponents of medical care would say: "Wait a minute, I don't think I quite bargained for this much. I don't quite think it is a disaster if blood does not run in the streets over this. I think we could sort this out in some more peaceful way."

I can remember times when some of our own people wondered if perhaps we should try to work out a different kind of plan. But we had been elected on a promise to put the plan in and we could not possibly allow what we thought was essentially a public relations campaign to thwart the desire of the electorate. We thought it was a good plan and would be good for Saskatchewan. We had a mandate to do it and an obligation to do it. If the whole thing collapsed around our ears, fine. We would be gone as a government, but we would be gone on a good cause.

So it was pretty intense. The premier and I were running negotiations, through third parties, while the minister of health was concentrating on keeping the health system running—getting doctors from Britain and so on. I was provincial treasurer and designated as the minister in charge of legal challenges. There were all sorts of things to contend with, including the possibility that in a wild stroke someone could get the courts to declare the Medical Care Insurance Act invalid. Some of the judges were violently opposed to this program and some of them were not beyond politics from time to time, as I suspect they are not in the United States either.

The press was violently opposed to us—by that I mean the two major newspapers, the *Regina Leader Post* and the *Saskatoon Star Phoenix,* which still exist. Both of them are owned by the same family, descendants of Clifford Sifton, who was a Liberal federal cabinet minister. With the CCF in power, these papers were violently antigovernment. No Sifton paper had ever

supported the CCF or the NDP, federally or provincially, in
any election, ever.

We had two major private television stations, CKCK in
Regina and CFQC in Saskatoon. The two dailies and the Regina TV station were all owned by the Siftons. The Saskatoon
station was owned by another family, equally right wing. Only
two families monopolized the two major private television stations and the only two dailies that mattered.

These were hard-line, right-wing papers, and in Regina
they had a particularly hard-line, right-wing editor. During the
dispute leading up to it and during the strike itself, they departed
from any and all principles of journalism and simply ran a paper
that campaigned against the medical care plan. If the news was
not good, they did a survey and announced the results. They
would sit down, pick twenty names, and call these people. What
do you know? The people they called were opposed to the plan.
It was really quite a shocking performance that went effectively
unchallenged — except by us — until after the strike started.

Once that happened, the place was flooded with reporters
from everywhere. I think it was about nine days into the strike
when the first editorial appeared in the Winnipeg paper saying
something like: "There is a strike going on and here is the news
about the strike. But we think you also should know what the
Saskatchewan newspapers are doing with this strike. Our reporters do not feel they are covering the same strike as the Saskatchewan newspapers."

The Saskatchewan newspapers began to say, "These outside reporters do not understand." This was kind of fun for us
in a way. We thought this was just splendid. Here we had some
of the best reporters in Canada and the United States being told
by these local reporters they did not understand something. The
papers in Saskatchewan did not command the best reporters.
It was like someone from the *Podunk Times,* or whatever, telling
the *New York Times* reporters they did not understand issues in
Ohio or Indiana. It was not a promising line to pursue.

I wrote a piece on this in which I documented my case.
It was called "Press Coverage and the Medicare Dispute" and
was published in the *Queen's Quarterly.* [1] I do not think anyone even

now challenges that the press coverage by the local Saskatchewan press, particularly the newspapers, was just outrageous.
The weeklies were just unbelievable. Some of them were owned
by people who were all upset because their doctor was going
to go away. They just knew this was true because that's what
their doctor was telling them. You can't do much about a weekly
in a situation like that, but the dailies should have been responsible and they were not. Everybody knew they were against us.

I remember one incident during the time the "Keep Our
Doctors" committee was running such a hard-line campaign saying the people were going to lose their doctors and the CCF
did not care. There appeared on a sidewalk in downtown Regina, in red paint, the slogan: "Doctors Get Out. Vote CCF."
It was obviously designed to suggest we wanted the doctors in
practice at the time to get out of medical care and leave town.
By a very odd stroke, the police apprehended and charged the
two people who were painting the sidewalk in this way. One
of them was a prominent member and the other an officer of
the competing Liberal Party organization. We hired a lawyer
to go down and try to say something to the judge about what
was happening. The judge just said, "Sorry, I am hearing these
people on the charges of defacing the sidewalk and I am not
interested in political parties." He was quite right in that, of
course, but we thought we would get a little altercation going.
We told our story to the reporters who were there, but the *Leader*
would not publish it.

When we asked why, they said something about libel. So
then we made up an ad, but they would not print it either. And
so we then put out a little leaflet with this information on it.
It was kind of a nice little story, but the *Leader* was having none
of it. They did run the picture of the mark on the sidewalk, and
they may have run the fact that two people were convicted. But
they were not having any part of our attempt to draw attention
to who did it.

It was pretty hardball.

Anyway, about eight or nine days into the strike we started
to get real coverage. The *Leader* and the *Star* kept to their ways
for the first few days, reporting all deaths and suggesting they

were a result of the doctors' strike, no matter what the individual circumstances were. They talked about trouble in hospitals,
beds being closed and people sent home sick, that sort of thing.
But once the other reporters came in, we began to get relief.
The Winnipeg papers were not only reporting the strike differently, they were beginning to question the way the Saskatchewan media were reporting it. By about the twelfth day, the
Leader's coverage was toned down a bit.

Things started coming together when I got a telephone
call from Donald MacPherson, whom I had known for some
time. He is about my age and we were in a Kinsman Club
together in Regina, something sort of like a junior Rotary Club,
a service club you cannot be in unless you are under forty. He
felt he could talk to me on behalf of the doctors.

This was around the middle of July, and I think the leaders
of the doctors' group were starting to think: "If this goes on until the end of July, our troops are going to come back and they
are going to open up their offices and we will not be able to hold
them. So we better make a settlement."

In a startling way, the President of the College of Physicians asked to speak to the annual convention of CCF of Saskatchewan, which happened to be meeting in Saskatoon. He,
in effect, laid down terms that were so close to what we could
accept that it was clear an agreement was near.

The negotiations took place in Saskatoon and what we
came up with was known as the Saskatoon Agreement. Woodrow
Lloyd, the premier, and I were holed up with a half dozen or
so others in the Bessborough Hotel, and the doctors were holed
up a couple of blocks away in that medical office tower that had
the "For Sale" sign out front. The sign had come down by now.

We had not consulted Lord Taylor before, but now we
called on him to come over from England to negotiate. He was
a Labour life peer and a physician with a good knowledge of
the British Health Service. He knew its weaknesses and was not
a wild advocate of it. And he was a showman par excellence.
All he wanted was expenses and one week of fishing to handle
the negotiations.

Taylor was going back and forth in his car, always parking

in the middle of the "No Parking" zone outside the hotel and putting a piece of House of Lords stationery in the window. He was quite a character.

He would say, "I am getting tired, I can't go on." He would put on this routine with us and then do the same thing with the doctors.

But eventually he pulled together an agreement.

Despite the intensity of that first year, Medicare was gone as an issue in Saskatchewan by 1964. We accused the Liberals, who had fought us so bitterly, of planning to dismantle it if they were elected. They swore on sixteen Bibles they were not going to dismantle it, and they did not. By 1964, it would have been politically unwise to say you were going to dismantle Medicare. By 1967, it would have been sheer and utter folly.

It was our issue, and now it's not an issue. The professionals among our political opponents always accuse us of trying to run another election on Medicare, and our pros respond that "we certainly damn well will if we can, if we have Medicare at risk again."

But they'll never give us an opening on that, because every poll you run shows that the public trusts us on Medicare and does not trust them on Medicare. If there is a perception that something is wrong with Medicare, that somehow it is threatened, then the voters will trust us to see that it is preserved. I am afraid that after twenty-five years, the voters do not really remember where it came from. But for a fair number of years, we were able to conjure up the possibility that someone was out there to torpedo Medicare.

We did lose power in that election in 1964, but not because of Medicare. The fact that they had a hard-driving new leader, the fact that we had lost the highly charismatic Douglas, and the fact that we had been in power twenty years allowed the party to fall victim to a coalition of forces. The party got more votes in 1964 than it got in 1960, because of the decline of two of the smaller parties, but the Liberal Party was able to get about one-half percent more votes than we did and the seat configuration was such that they were able to form a new provincial government.

Our support of the medical plan contributed to our 1964 defeat to the extent that it stirred up so much controversy and helped energize the Liberal Party. But it was not the reason for the Liberals gaining power, as evidenced by the fact that they did not change Medicare in any significant way in their seven years of office. We regained power in 1971 and I became premier.

Notwithstanding the opposition of the doctors and all the controversy and the beating we took in the 1962 federal election, the medical care plan soon enough was thought by almost everyone in Saskatchewan to be a good thing — not right away, but after it got in place and demonstrated that it worked. We had this operational plan that served as a model.

John Diefenbaker, a sort of populist Tory from Saskatchewan who was prime minister in the late 1950s and early 1960s, concluded that "we should be looking at this for Canada" and appointed a Royal Commission, headed by his old friend from Saskatchewan — Emmett Hall — to study the matter. Hall knew the Saskatchewan plan worked, and so he recommended a national plan that is really quite similar to the Saskatchewan version.

Then we had a Liberal prime minister, Lester Pearson, who succeeded Diefenbaker. He wanted to make a mark for himself and thought this would be a good way to do it. So he turned to the deputy minister of National Health and Welfare to flesh out details of the plan he was going to put forward. That happened to be Al Johnson, who had been a deputy provincial treasurer in Saskatchewan when I was provincial treasurer in 1962, and who was perhaps the leading public servant we had in the province. He left after we were knocked out of power in 1964, went to Ottawa, and soon became deputy minister of National Health and Welfare.

Johnson just pulled the Saskatchewan plan off the shelf. He knew the plan very well because he was instrumental in drafting it, and away we went.

First there was Diefenbaker and the accident of him appointing Hall, who recommended something very close to the Saskatchewan plan. Then we had Pearson, a member of the Liberal Party, turning to Johnson, another accident.

Out of all of this came a proposal for a national scheme

that looked really remarkably like the Saskatchewan scheme because the actors all came out of this tradition. This was just an accident of history.

But the real key was Lester Pearson's willingness to go forward with it and his willingness to go forward without the approval of provincial governments.

By this time, the provinces were beginning to say, "You should not bring any more of these cost-sharing programs in without prior consultation with us because it puts us in a terrible bind. We have to take them and distort all our spending priorities, or leave big chunks of money on the federal table, which we cannot do because our people are paying the taxes that provide that money."

They could not have gotten these provinces to agree to it. Quebec would acquiesce but could not possibly agree in advance to a program with so many federal strings on, for a host of reasons. But they really needed a scheme like this. They would grumble, but they would acquiesce and be happy to have it. Ontario would acquiesce and be happy with it. They are the wealthiest province, and essentially they put out more of the money than they get back. But they are used to it. They would grumble a bit, like California, but they are used to putting more into the pot than they get out.

So Pearson didn't bother trying to get a federal provincial agreement because that would have taken a decade. It was a courageous move that raised a little flack, but he just went with it.

He was succeeded by Pierre Trudeau in 1968. Trudeau used the famous line "there will be no more Medicares" as a way of declaring there would no more major cost-sharing programs announced by the federal government without significant prior consultation with the provinces.

There was no fight when Pearson moved, other than a little squabble on federal-provincial issues. But there was no fight from the medical profession. It was all over. That battle had been fought, and won, in Saskatchewan.

I think this was partly because the plan was not nearly as bad as the doctors thought it would be, and partly because they took the position that they would control its worst excesses and would lose an all-out fight anyway. It was a shrewd judgment.

The Ontario doctors ran a short strike a few years ago when the Ontario government passed a law against extra billing and coinsurance. But it was a disastrous failure. They had no public support at all. The Ontario papers ran cartoons of doctors; I can remember one of three or four doctors with their white coats and stethoscopes driving a Rolls Royce, singing "Solidarity Forever."

The government was successful in arguing that the doctors were just striking for more money. The public perception is that doctors do very well, thank you very much, and that whoever may need to strike for more money, it is not doctors.

In our case, in 1962, I think the perception was not so much that doctors made masses of money—except maybe for the specialists—but that doctors simply should not strike. It was a moral position, that doctors have no right to withdraw their services from patients.

Interestingly enough, the plan helped doctors financially. The specialists' income probably didn't go up as much, but the general practitioners did much, much better. There is no question that it was an absolute bonanza for the doctors—so much so that if you had said five years later you were going to do away with the whole plan, I think you would have had a strike the other way.

One little problem we had that probably will be significant in the United States was with the trade unions, who had already had medical insurance and who felt that now they were going to have to pay extra taxes to pay for this insurance they already had. As they saw it, there were going to be very substantial savings to their employers and they were going to get none of it. They would say: "Look at the last bargaining session. We actually took less money in order for the employer to pay the medical care insurance premiums, and now you are going to take all of this load off the employer and we are going to get none of it. That's dirty pool."

What we did was say the employer had to ascertain the amount being paid in medical care insurance on behalf of each employee and add that amount to the paycheck until the next bargaining. After that, they could decide in negotiations how to handle it. The theory was that the employers would be no better or worse off because they were not going to have to pay for insurance and the employees would be no worse off because the cash value of it would be transferred to them. At the time of the next bargaining, they were going to have to sort that out between themselves. This was a temporary addition to the pay package, and whether it was permanent or whether it was split or whether it was converted into some additional and other benefits, such as dental benefits — that was for the employers and employees to work out.

The employers did not like that. They said, "Look, we are going to have to pay extra taxes, too, and we are going to have to transfer all this value over to the employee."

We basically said, "We cannot split hairs any further." We were essentially financing this by a 2 percent increase in sales taxes — from 3 percent to 5 percent — and the big load of that would fall on consumers, although some employers would have to pay. We knew some of the employers would be disadvantaged during the transition period, but we just could not get down to legislating a degree of arithmetic detail that would take care of every situation. Our idea was that they would just have to sort it out in the next negotiations, because this is the best compromise we can make.

It was a political problem because it was raised by people who ordinarily supported us, the trade unions.

They are natural philosophical allies, but not always as natural as they should be because many people in organized labor are on the upper end of the socioeconomic ladder. It is the unorganized labor that needs this thing most, or the very ill-organized.

This is something that certainly will arise in the United States, because you have that enormous number of people who have coverage through their employers that was negotiated under union contracts.

Let me make another sidebar comment. There was virtually no commercial health insurance industry in Saskatchewan when we put our plan in place. There were a few small insurance plans run mostly by doctors to facilitate their getting paid, and they made an effort to be involved in the settlement arrangement. But they were not a significant factor.

The Saskatoon agreement that ended the Medicare dispute provided that doctors could be paid by sending their bills to the Medical Care Insurance Commission or to an approved health insurance agency if the patient was a member of one. But they would get the same amount of money either way, and it would come from the government. This was largely a face-saving device for those doctors who did not want to deal with the government, who would have nothing to do with socialized medicine or state medicine or whatever epithet they had learned to pronounce. These doctor-sponsored health care insurance agencies would gather up all the bills, send them to the government, and get one check back. They would then divide the money and send the payments on to the doctors. But this was an extra step that had little real utility for anyone.

The great bulk of the doctors took a posture of "we've got to live with this, so let's get on with it." It worked like a charm. They sent their bills straight to the government and their checks came back in the mail, in nice large amounts. They thought this was great.

Because of the size of the commercial health insurance industry, anyone trying to implement a program similar to ours in the United States undoubtedly would have much larger problems along these lines than we did.

CHAPTER 6

Delivering and Financing Long Term Care in Canada's Ten Provinces

Rosalie A. Kane

Canada offers some valuable lessons for the United States in organization and delivery of long term care.[1] At the very minimum, the Canadian experience illustrates the art of the possible at a time when pessimism prevails in the United States regarding genuine, far-reaching long term care reform. Conventional wisdom in the United States holds that universal coverage of acute care for all Americans cannot be afforded — and that adding long term care would be unthinkable. Further, although many recognize that the heavy tilt toward public financing of nursing home care, rather than home-based care, runs counter to the preferences and needs of most users of long term care, conventional wisdom suggests that the costs of providing subsidized benefits for long term care in the community would be uncontrollable.

In sharp contrast, there is a fifteen-year history of both these reforms in parts of Canada. First, there has been a move from a spend-down, means-tested public benefit for nursing home care to a universal benefit — albeit one that is cost shared with the users. Second, there has been a move toward offering a wide array of long term care services in the community as well as in nursing homes. U.S. policy makers would do well to study the Canadian experience, because it provides perhaps the best international comparison to the United States.

Both are industrialized nations with federal governments
that have the greatest taxing power among all governmental
levels. In both systems, money is distributed from the central
government to the states — in Canada's case to the provinces —
by a variety of methods, including block grants. The state and
provincial governments zealously defend their autonomous rights
in both countries, and some states or provinces are wealthier
than others. The age distribution is similar in the two, although
the U.S. population is aging a little faster. And the delivery of
health care is markedly similar: fee-for-service physicians, different types of hospitals, and both for-profit and not-for-profit nursing homes.

Moreover, Canadian and U.S. citizens share much in
their historical and contemporary cultures, and both countries
contend with large land masses and an uneven distribution of
the population. In Canada, there are vast underpopulated northern areas, with the population concentrated near the U.S. border.
Although not as extreme, the United States similarly has a huge
region of Western states where the sparse population presents
far different health delivery challenges than those encountered
along the teeming coasts and in the industrial regions of the
Midwest.

Long term care financing and delivery were similar in
Canada and the United States as recently as two decades ago.
The nursing home predominated as the form of service receiving public financing, but residents of nursing homes needed to
be poor before they could receive benefits. Despite means and
asset testing for nursing home financial assistance, at least half
of the costs of nursing home care fell to the provinces or the
states, which chafed under growing and seemingly uncontrollable expenditures. The home care sector was underdeveloped,
as it remains in the United States.

Unlike acute care, long term care still is not part of the
universal health insurance program in Canada and thus remains
largely a provincial matter.

However, federal funds are available through the per capita extended care block grant, initiated in 1977, and through
federal cost sharing for poor clients under the Canada Assistance

Program. But great discretion is left to the provincial governments in how to administer their programs. Each is left to determine the nature of services, eligibility standards, reimbursement policies, and the extent of consumer cost sharing.

Predictably, this results in wide variations among the provinces in the shape of nursing home care, as well as home- and community-based care.

Nursing Home Care

The Canadian federal government acted in 1973 to clarify the continuum of institutionally based health care, releasing a five-level classification scheme.

Level 1 is residential, Level 2 is extended care, Level 3 is chronic hospital, Level 4 is rehabilitation, and Level 5 is acute hospital.

Extended care in Canada is analogous to skilled and intermediate nursing home care in the United States, and residential care is analogous to board and care. The terminology for the other three levels — acute hospital, rehabilitation, and chronic hospital — is roughly the same in both countries.

In Canada, acute hospital, rehabilitation, and chronic hospital are covered automatically for the whole country as part of comprehensive coverage under the universal national hospital assurance. All but three provinces insure nursing home care at the extended care and residential level, which is to say they make nursing home care available to all people regardless of income or assets, albeit with consumers required to pay part of the costs. The three without universally insured nursing home care — New Brunswick, Nova Scotia, and Prince Edward Island — have less than 5 percent of the country's population.

Prior to 1970, the Canadian provinces subsidized nursing home care for the poor, but people with financial means were expected to pay for their care as long as their resources would permit. Like state governments in the United States today, provincial governments found that they were paying more than half the total nursing home bill, with little control over usage or quality.

Ontario and Manitoba began insuring nursing home care
in the 1970s, and the federal Established Programs Financing
Act introduced a per capita block grant to each province, called
the *extended care grant,* in 1977. Initially fixed at $20 per capita,
with an automatic annual escalator for inflation, this grant was
designed to permit provinces the flexibility to go beyond hospital care with less expensive and perhaps more desirable forms
of care such as home care, nursing home care, and other special programs for targeted groups. This gave provinces the incentive to attempt universal nursing home insurance, and most
began that program in the late 1970s and early 1980s.

Despite provincial variation, the rudiments of the nursing home insurance program are constant. Functionally im-
paired residents are eligible for nursing home care regardless
of income, assets, or age. But the care is not free. Typically,
the resident pays a fixed sum equal to about a third of the daily
rate for so-called "ward accommodations," which can be a four-
bed room but often is a two-bed room. The consumer payment
is fixed so the poorest resident can afford it and be left with a
rather generous allowance for personal spending. The consumer
payment and the personal allowance rise annually with the cost-
of-living index. But the personal allowance is more than twice
the comfort allowance permitted nursing home residents by even
the most generous states in the "spend-down" U.S. Medicaid
system.

Because Canadian nursing home residents do not have
to impoverish themselves before qualifying for government assistance, most can afford extra amenities, including single rooms.
Facilities are strictly controlled in the amount of additional
charges permitted for single rooms. Ontario is considering a
proposal — to be reviewed in public hearings over the next few
years — that would increase consumer copays and adjust the
amount to income.

The basic nursing home rate is negotiated annually between the provincial government and the provincial nursing
home association. Nursing homes are expected to care for residential (and, in particular, extended care) patients. Some provinces have expanded this to create other levels of long term care

need. In those cases, nursing homes are reimbursed at different rates for the different levels of care.

Nursing homes in Canada are operated on both a for-profit and a nonprofit basis, although the proportion of nonprofit homes is much higher in Canada than in the United States. Nonprofit homes, generally owned by sectarian groups or municipalities, often are known in Canada as homes for the aging. Their history was one of providing residential programs for the poor regardless of their health status. But by the time provinces introduced universal extended care benefits, many residents in homes for the aging had, in fact, aged to the point that they qualified for the new health-based benefit. The use pattern has changed over the last few decades so that fewer well elderly people enter homes for the aging, partly because of better income maintenance and because of better housing and home care programs. Extended care sections in homes for the aging consequently have expanded, and many people with disabilities now are admitted directly into most homes for the aging. Data from Ontario suggest that acuity levels are higher among residents of homes for the aging than of the for-profit nursing homes.

Ownership patterns of nursing homes vary from province to province. Ontario, the most populous province, has two sectors of institutional long term care: an almost completely for-profit nursing home sector that in 1984 housed more than 21,000 people in 332 homes and a nonprofit homes-for-the-aging sector that in 1982 housed 30,000 people in 180 homes, more than half of which were in extended care beds.[2]

The provinces have tended to make distinctions in the way they reimburse homes, depending on their ownership. Historically, the provincial government covered the operating deficit for the nonprofit homes, virtually underwriting the differences between the consumer payments and the facilities' expenses. For-profit homes, by contrast, were paid a fixed per diem. British Columbia modified that scheme some years ago so the two sectors would be treated more equitably. The issue is highly contentious in Ontario, with the nursing homes claiming unfair treatment and the homes for the aged arguing that the for-profit homes skim the market. A task force is considering reform, including a possible reimbursement system adjusted by case mix for both sectors.

Regulation of nursing homes in Canada is much less rigorous and bureaucratized than in the United States, but Canadians are far from sanguine about the quality of their nursing homes. The facilities are licensed and inspected by the provincial governments, again with variation from province to province. As in the United States, the perceived quality varies from region to region. In Ontario, where for-profit homes are most numerous, an active grass-roots organization called Concerned Friends of Ontario Nursing Home Residents has clamored for more resources and better quality control.

Provinces control the supply of nursing home beds in various ways. In Ontario, for example, the province calls for competitive bids for the "right to build" when it determines that additional beds are needed in a particular region. The applicants do not compete on price, which is fixed, but rather on their track record for quality and on their promised programs and amenities. Critics argue that the supply of extended care beds in Ontario is inadequate and that many people therefore are forced to use private rest homes, which are not covered at all under the Extended Care Benefit.

Although most nursing home care in Canada is in freestanding facilities, many hospitals also have long term care beds. Particularly in rural areas, hospitals have been encouraged to develop long term care units for long-stay patients. In cities with geriatric medicine programs, geriatricians may exert control over hospital beds where patients can go after their acute phase is over. Unless designated as Level 3 or Level 4 (chronic hospital or rehabilitation), care in these beds is reimbursed at nursing home rates in the hospital's global budget and the consumer is responsible for a daily copayment, just as in a freestanding nursing home.

In sum, all but 5 percent of Canadians are insured against the cost of nursing home care. They are not required to "spend down" their financial resources but do have to pay a flat daily rate, which some consider "the cheapest rent in town." Canada's greatest progress in caring for its elderly in need of long term care has been to successfully underwrite the cost of nursing home care — as opposed to fundamentally changing the nature of the living environment or the services in nursing homes. That alone, however, is no mean accomplishment.

Home and Community-based Care

As with nursing home care, Canadian provinces vary in the way they handle home care services.

Programs for acute care in the home generally were implemented in the 1970s or earlier as part of the universal health insurance programs. These were viewed in part as "hospital replacement" services and were operated by local health departments of the Victorian Order of Nurses, a nonprofit agency analogous to the Visiting Nurse Associations in the United States. The programs did not develop their present comprehensive characteristics until much later.

In 1974, Manitoba became the first province to develop a fully rounded home care program in which service levels were based on assessments of functional abilities and no physician referral or supervision was required. Nurse and social work teams in district health offices do the assessments and authorize and manage the service. British Columbia implemented both its institutional long term care benefits and its home care benefits in 1978, establishing a continuing care program for assessment and allocation of services in each local health department. British Columbia recognizes five levels of long term care. A reimbursement level for nursing homes has been established, and a maximum amount of home care set for each level.

Ontario, on the other hand, put its home care programs in place piecemeal. Acute care at home was introduced as a health insurance benefit in 1968. So-called "chronic home care" had been tried on a pilot basis in a few of the province's thirty-eight health districts as early as 1965. However, the phase in of chronic home care was gradual, and it was not until 1984 that metropolitan Toronto, the most populous district, was authorized to offer the service on a regular basis. Both acute and chronic home care programs require referral from a physician and ongoing involvement of a registered nurse. In 1986, the province authorized six Integrated Homemaker Programs—sometimes called "homemaker only programs"—on a pilot basis. Although administered by the same home health system as the others, these programs offer homemaker and meal benefits to those who do not otherwise need professional assistance.

Fees usually are not charged for the nursing part of the home care programs. Nova Scotia is an exception and imposes some fees for nursing services. However, the provinces vary widely in fee policies for homemaker services. Newfoundland and New Brunswick have no charges at all, Quebec charges for meals and transportation, and Prince Edward Island, Nova Scotia, Ontario, Saskatchewan, and British Columbia all charge according to a sliding scale based on income. In Alberta, all home support services except meals are free for the first two weeks and then are billed on a sliding scale ranging from $3 a visit to $300 a month. All provinces report they recover very little money for the home care services.

Although no provinces limit health-related home care by age, four limit the more socially oriented services to older people. Many provinces have a history of home support programs specifically for the old—such as meal and friendly-visit programs staffed by volunteers—that originated as social service programs. These often continue alongside the more medically oriented programs.

Like the benefits provided, the organization structure of the provincial home care programs varies.

British Columbia and Saskatchewan both have created organizational entities called *Continuing Care Programs* that are responsible for administering both nursing home and home care and for controlling access to both. But the responsibility for home care and institutional long term care is split in Manitoba, New Brunswick, Newfoundland, Nova Scotia, Prince Edward Island, and Quebec—sometimes involving several different provincial ministries.[3]

Two provinces and the vast, underpopulated northern territories have not developed separate home care programs.

Provincial benefit and administrative differences notwithstanding, the Canadian home-based services always include visiting nurse services, personal care, and homemaking. All provinces with programs also consider a comprehensive assessment, such as is done by a case manager or care coordinator, as a pivotal service. Physical therapy, occupational therapy, pulmonary therapy, and social work often are included but are not always available in rural areas. Home equipment and supplies are made available in all provinces, and the use of such equipment often is coordinated by the home care program. Day care also is coordinated in some cases by the home care managers, and most programs try to organize respite services either at home, at inpatient facilities, or at day-care centers. Meal services sometimes are arranged by the home care programs. A handyman service for snow shoveling, yard work, and heavy chores is considered distinct from homemaking in some programs.

The actual delivery of services essentially comes down to two methods: provinces deliver the services themselves by hiring nurses and other personnel to work at the local level, or they contract with other organizations to provide the services. In fact, both mechanisms often are used side by side, and each province has evolved its own pattern of which services to deliver directly and which to let out to contract. In some provinces, the Victorian Order of Nurses (VON) coordinates short-term acute home care and provides nursing services, at least in large cities. But many provinces have moved toward maintaining their own nursing staffs. The recent pattern in Manitoba, for example, was to use the VON for acute home care in Winnipeg and staff nurses for all other services. Four provinces, including Manitoba and populous Quebec, employ homemakers and personal care attendants directly, while the others contract with local agencies. The Red Cross is a dominant homemaking provider in much of Canada, including Ontario. But for-profit homemaking agencies also are found, especially in the cities.

At the local level, case management is integral to most of the long term care programs. Typically, the care coordinator is a nurse or a social worker who performs an assessment and makes a care plan. Generally speaking, the Canadian programs, like case-managed community care programs in the

United States, will not authorize a care program in the community that would cost more than care for the same person in a nursing home. Exceptions might be short-term care for a terminally ill person, or care that substitutes for a hospital admission. But the decision about where to provide the care is secondary to the decision about the level of care needed. Each level theoretically can be accommodated at home if enough volunteered family care is available.

In British Columbia, the care coordinators also authorize nursing home care, assist the person in finding the nursing home of his or her choosing, and continue to monitor the level of care needed. If the person must enter a facility immediately and there is no vacancy in the preferred facility, he or she may be put on a waiting list and be transferred to the preferred nursing home when space opens up.

In Manitoba, the care coordinators do not monitor clients after they enter nursing homes. But in Manitoba, nobody can be put on a waiting list for a nursing home unless the case is reviewed formally by a multidisciplinary panel, usually headed by a geriatrician. The case manager must present full information, including data from the client's primary care physician. The panel system serves as a safeguard against hasty decisions. Sometimes the panel elects to refer the client for a full geriatric assessment and short-range treatment before authorizing a nursing home.

In Ontario, care coordination is less systematic, although case managers do work out of each home care program. Ontario developed mechanisms called *Placement Coordination Services,* which are voluntary arrangements among hospitals, nursing homes, and homes for the aged in a particular locality to coordinate waiting lists for nursing homes.

Although the Canadian provincial long term care programs differ in detail, more striking is what they have in common:

- Universal entitlement for nursing home care
- Affordable consumer copays for nursing home care
- Eligibility for nursing home care and home care unrestricted by income, assets, or age
- A wide array of services available at home, including high-

tech medically oriented home care, hospice care, short-term "acute" home care following hospitalization, long-range personal care to meet chronic health needs, and socially oriented home care

Government benefits generally pay the first dollar for long term care, both institutional and home based. Those with means can use their own resources to add a greater level of service, sometimes hiring the same home care personnel to give extra service. This is the opposite strategy from the one in the United States, where consumers pay the first dollar — with government benefits becoming available only when their resources are low or exhausted. In both systems, however, some form of case management or care coordination is used to allocate services and some form of functional assessment usually governs service levels.

Long term care costs in Canada are considered as part of the nation's total health care costs, which are widely acknowledged to be less per capita and less as a proportion of the gross domestic product (GDP) than health care costs in the United States — even though the U.S. calculations most frequently used for comparison do not include long term care expenses.

Utilization of Canadian home-based services appears to be manageable, and provincial officials report that once programs stabilized and caseloads accrued, there was no groundswell of inappropriate demand for services. Family members continue to provide care for their relatives at home, and the programs are organized around the expectation that such family involvement will continue. Nonetheless, eligibility is not limited to people with family members, nor are family members required to give a particular service for their relative to be eligible for government assistance.

Despite the encouraging news on utilization and costs, provincial governments remain concerned about the growth of expenditures in these programs. Studies have been commissioned to examine ways to make community care more efficient, and one recent study in Manitoba recommended sweeping changes. Indeed, home care programs appear to be more vulnerable than nursing home programs to the restrictive tendencies of cost-conscious governments. Although home care costs less for a person who can function in that setting than putting the same individual in a nursing home, the home care programs seem to policy makers to be more amenable to cutting than nursing home programs.

Moreover, there are ever-present tensions in Canadian federalism, with periodic attempts to reduce the federal contribution for a number of health and human service programs and, therefore, to increase the disparity in provisions among wealthier and poorer provinces.

Provinces either already rely on, or are attempting to encourage, a range of volunteer community support services such as friendly-visiting, transportation, meal delivery, and even cleaning services. When such programs are available at the local level from nonprofit organizations, most provinces have a policy of not replicating those services at government expense. The emphasis on encouraging nonprofit providers presumably is based on an assumption that such service is likely to be free or cost little. Case managers in some jurisdictions are frustrated because they believe the nonprofit supportive organizations are inadequate to meet the tasks.

In a review of Canadian home care programs, Robert L. Kane and I found that the provinces, varied as they are in programs and circumstances, were grappling with similar questions about their maturing home care programs.[4] One issue concerned how far to go with the delivery of sophisticated, intensive, and highly technical services at home. Given the high level of personnel costs, the question was whether such high-tech home care was justified when the effort would do little more than replace hospital admissions or shorten hospital stays.

At the other end of the technological continuum, some provinces are struggling over the extent to which housekeeping and other "low-tech" home-based services should be part of a universal benefit for health care. Provincial officials all seem to agree that intensive health care at home that replaces hospital care, skilled rehabilitation services at home, and even personal care for maintenance of the chronically ill at home fall under universal health insurance principles. On the other hand, there is some emerging consensus that socially oriented services such as housekeeping should fall outside health programs and, therefore, should be financed by combinations of private payments and subsidies for the poor. The practical question is where to draw the line and how to avoid fragmentation and duplication at the local service delivery level.

Another issue concerns whether a principle of equivalence between nursing home care and home care should be maintained, or whether care should be viewed on a continuum — with efforts made to determine when home care is "appropriate" and when a "higher level" is needed. Some provinces take the stance that the choice should be up to the client, bearing in mind that the province will not pay more for home care than for a nursing home. Others are trying to develop the continuum notion.

All the provinces have had difficulty staffing remote rural areas, particularly for home care, and all have developed flexible patterns, improvising when an entire health team cannot be mustered. Except for remote areas, however, it does not appear that Canadian provinces experience a labor shortage of people willing to serve as paraprofessional home care providers. This may be partly because such workers tend to enjoy much better wages and benefits than their counterparts in the United States.

Given the necessity of oversimplification when presenting an overview of widely disparate programs (and given their constant evolution), they nonetheless may safely be characterized as efficient, popular with the public, and readily affordable.

The Canadian programs can and will be improved and modified. But Canadian citizens already have come to take for granted a level of long term care benefits far exceeding anything yet contemplated in the United States by any but the most farsighted and idealistic individuals.

CHAPTER 7

Serving Elderly Patients:
The Benefits of Integrated Long Term Care in British Columbia

Paul Pallan

Elsie is a widow in her mid eighties, living in Victoria, B.C. She fell during an early morning walk and was taken to a hospital emergency room with a broken left arm and abrasions on her leg.

But Elsie didn't want to stay in the hospital. She wanted to recover at home, where she could take care of her cat. The emergency room doctor agreed that she would be okay in her own home if adequate help was available. But she had no relatives nearby and no friends young enough or sprightly enough to help her.

So the physician contacted the Quick Response Team (QRT) in Victoria, which was established in 1986 to prevent unnecessary hospitalization for the frail elderly.

The physician outlined Elsie's condition to the team liaison nurse: her arm would have to be supported by a sling, her bandages needed changing every day, and she needed physiotherapy and occupational therapy to regain full use of her arm.

The QRT nurse assigned a home support worker to live with Elsie, explaining what signs and symptoms to look for, how to care for her arm, and how much pain medication she needed.

Next, a physiotherapist visited Elsie's home to size up the situation. She ordered a special commode from an equipment loan service, to make it easier for Elsie to get up and down. She created an exercise regime for her, explaining to the home support worker how to adjust the program as Elsie improved and was able to do more.

Within five days, she was able to move around her home with little assistance and was placed in a community home nursing care program, in which someone visited once a day to check on her arm and change the dressing on her leg wounds.

As Elsie recovered and regained more and more independence, the level of the community support services decreased gradually with her decreasing needs.

Jane, also an elderly woman living alone in Victoria, was left with partial paralysis on her left side after suffering a stroke. She, too, wanted to recover at home, not in the hospital.

Enter the Quick Response Team.

A QRT nurse and occupational therapist visited Jane to assess what sort of help she would need during recovery. They noted some memory problems, weakness in her left leg, and a lack of movement in her left arm. She would need help just to move around and wash and dress herself. A neighbor could help with such things as picking up a few groceries, but there were no family or friends available to stay with Jane and provide the kind of assistance she would need to remain safely in her own home.

So the team set up a care plan suited to Jane's needs. The nurse contacted a home support agency, arranging for a worker to stay with Jane and help her with personal care and getting around her house.

A wheelchair was brought in so Jane could move around her house more easily—and even get out to her garden—and an occupational therapist visited every day to help her learn how to bathe and dress using only her right side.

A physiotherapist also saw Jane every day for the first few days to instruct her and her home support worker on the best positions for her left arm and leg. She showed Jane how to move her paralyzed arm, giving her exercises to improve strength and coordination. She also wrote down some simple exercises she could practice on her own.

The team nurse visited regularly to monitor Jane's vital

signs and medications and organized the medicine so she could manage them herself.

As Jane improved to the point where she no longer required full-time home support, a worker was supplied two hours a day, three days a week to assist with housework, meals, and bathing.

The Quick Response Team worked with Jane until she could walk on her own in the house, manage the stairs, and get around outside her home with the help of a cane. The team then referred her to the outpatient department of the local rehabilitation hospital for continuing therapy.

Bob, eighty-four, was hospitalized after falling in his house. Although he was not really hurt by the fall, Bob's doctor noted that he had fallen several times in recent months. While in the hospital, he also was diagnosed with diabetes that required daily injections of insulin.

Bob's daughter Lynn was worried. She had seen his condition deteriorate since her mother's recent death and was concerned about his safety, since another fall could be dangerous. And she fretted about his poor eating habits.

Lynn thought it would be better for her father to move into a facility where he would be under constant supervision by a professional staff, but Bob wanted to return to his own home and the belongings that had meant so much to him all his life — and where his deceased wife's memory was a comforting presence.

A social worker from the Quick Response Team described available home care services to Bob and Lynn, and they all agreed that Bob could manage to stay at home with appropriate help from the provincial long term care program.

The social worker talked to Bob's doctor about the possibility of an early discharge from the hospital; the doctor agreed to the discharge on the condition that Bob would receive adequate home care services.

Again, the Quick Response Team social worker arranged for Bob's care after his return home. She and a nurse met Bob when he arrived home from the hospital and discussed his care plan. The condition of Bob's home indicated that he had been having difficulty managing on his own for some time. Clearly, he needed help with laundry, cleaning, and meal preparation.

The social worker arranged for a home support worker to provide these services three days a week. She also arranged for Meals on Wheels to deliver hot meals regularly. A nutritionist was sent in to teach Bob about maintaining a balanced diet.

A nurse visited to check Bob's circulation and follow up on the training he got in the hospital on how to give himself insulin injections. She taught him more about his diabetes and checked to see that he was eating right.

An occupational therapist visited to check the safety of Bob's home to prevent future falls, recommending that he remove several scatter rugs and rearrange some of his furniture to reduce potential hazards.

During follow-up visits to his home, team members noticed that Bob was getting stronger and walking more steadily. At their suggestion, he agreed to have a telephone alert system installed in his home so immediate help would be available if he needed it.

As he improved, the home support service was gradually reduced to weekly visits to assist with cleaning and laundry. Meals on Wheels service, however, was increased to be sure that Bob continued to have a healthy diet. And Bob was encouraged to attend a government-funded activity center every week to get more involved and meet new people.

Although the real-life experiences of Elsie, Jane, and Bob illustrate the efficiency and sensitivity of the British Columbia approach to caring for people in need, the long term care systems there and in the other Canadian provinces are still evolving — particularly in contrast to the acute care systems that have been in place much longer.

The British Columbia long term care system really was only started in 1978. And in some Canadian provinces, long term care is still very much in the development stage.

Nonetheless, development of long term care programs is following the same principles that shaped Canada's acute care system.

The philosophy is to stress the independence of the individual first and foremost. Wherever possible, community-based services are emphasized as opposed to residential care. The concept of choice is very important in Canadian programs, and a multiplicity of services are offered so individuals can choose those most appropriate to their particular requirements.

Another fundamental goal, of course, is to maintain reasonable levels of access at reasonable cost.

The whole of the health care program in British Columbia is a managed system, and the long term care component does not exist in isolation. It is coordinated with the hospital system, the medical system, the drug-dispensing system, and so on. Perhaps most important, the government long term care system complements the varieties of informal care available: it is not intended to replace the informal assistance provided by friends and family.

British Columbia's provincial government recognized a growing need for a universal long term care program in the mid 1970s. Many residents needed long term care services, but the existing system required them to use virtually all of their personal resources before becoming eligible for government-sponsored care. This approach clearly was quite contrary to the general philosophy that health care was a universal right—the underpinning of the existing hospital and medical care programs already in existence and working well.

Faced with public pressure to introduce a universal program, the "conservative" Social Credit government recognized that the timing was right: not only would there be strong political support, but the federal government was modifying its arrangements with the provinces to provide a $20 per capita incentive to develop "extended health programs." The existing system already provided financial assistance to many low-income clients. In the new system, new clients would be expected to contribute toward their daily room and board costs—but only to the extent they were able to pay without impoverishing themselves. In some cases, they would pay extra for preferred accommodations.

In short, the overall financial consequence to the provincial governments of embarking on long term care programs would not be as traumatic as once feared.

As elsewhere in Canada, the long term care program in

British Columbia is managed by the province, which is responsible for bearing the cost of approved services, developing overall policies and legislation to support the various health programs, developing overall standards, and carrying out long-range planning.

More than 90 percent of the money paid out goes to "third-party" providers such as hospitals, physicians, long term care facilities, and homemaker agencies. These third parties are autonomous but, in exchange for being paid by the government, must abide by the legislation and policies established by the province.

While the system is operated by the province with provincial tax revenue, it also receives some money from the federal government in the form of transfer payments.

Any British Columbia resident over nineteen years of age is eligible for the program. (Younger people with chronic needs are taken care of in other programs.) The long term care system divides the province into twenty-one regions, each with long term care assessors, who are responsible for determining whether an individual is eligible for services and which services would most appropriately meet the person's needs. Any community of at least 2,000 to 3,000 residents typically has access to long term care assessment services.

As with Elsie, Jane, and Bob, when an individual first comes in contact with the long term care system, the assessor goes to the person's home for an interview — usually lasting about an hour — to assess the individual's need. It is particularly important that the interview be conducted in the person's home, sometimes with children or other family members present, because the assessor can see all of the environmental factors affecting that individual.

The assessor or case manager considers the individual's ability to manage activities of daily living, their health status and mental functioning, how well they can get around, their social functioning, and their financial position.

The assessor outlines the range of options available and determines the wishes of the individual and family in order to develop a care plan that is satisfactory to all.

In essence, the assessor becomes a case manager. Should the person be going into residential care? Or is care more appropriately provided through government-financed community resources, or even by an informal support network? What do the individual and family want?

Wherever possible, the assessor will promote the use of home support and community services and continued family involvement in meeting the client's requirements.

In some cases, the assessor will need additional medical information to make these decisions, and the patient's general practitioner may be called on to help. There are also places called short-stay assessment and treatment centers that can make determinations about complex medical issues affecting an individual. For example, a person might be displaying frequent mood changes that are affecting his or her mental state. The short-stay assessment and treatment center is staffed by physicians and other professionals who specialize in geriatric care. Through an inpatient admission, or on an outpatient basis, they may determine that the impact of multiple medications is contributing to the mood swings. Being able to deal with such a situation by an appropriate adjustment of medications may help avoid an unnecessary admission to a facility.

If the initial assessment indicates that a person has a problem with the activities of daily living, or some other chronic health problem, the client will be deemed qualified to receive care and can enter the system that provides access to a range of residential facilities and home support services. Residential facilities available include group homes, foster homes, and various types of chronic care homes. On the home support side, there are visiting homemakers, home care nurses, community-based physiotherapists, Meals on Wheels, and adult day-care centers.

The provincial government controls the assessment process and employs the staff that makes the determination of need. In a few health units, the assessors are hired by local municipalities, but these assessors are required to comply with provincial policies and procedures. Most of the services actually provided to care recipients are purchased by the province from private, third-party providers on a contract basis.

British Columbia has a population of over three million, of which 360,000 are over the age of sixty-five. (About 80 percent of long term care costs are attributable to people over sixty-five.)[1] The overall government cost of long term care services was $430 million in 1989–90.[2] That works out to a little more than $140 (Canadian) per capita. Even if you add in the cost of funding designated extended care units, or chronic care facilities, it's only slightly over $200 (Canadian) per capita—or about $4 a week per British Columbian. (That's less than U.S. $3.50.)

I find it striking that administrative costs alone for health care in the United States amount to about U.S. $95 per person per year, or about $115 (Canadian). British Columbians don't spend all that much more to fund our entire long term care program than Americans spend to cover just the administrative costs alone of your health care system.

Roughly 75 percent of the $430 million spent in British Columbia goes toward residential care. Something around $100 million is spent on home support services.[3] The actual program management costs are about $4 million, or 1 percent of the long term care budget.

The British Columbia long term care system operates on a safety net principle that holds that no individual will be charged more than they are able to pay for any services received.

Essentially, an individual pays $20 (Canadian) per day for residential care. That $20 represents 85 percent of the minimum pension level for anybody above the age of sixty-five in British Columbia. After an individual has paid the residential care bill, he or she will have about $150 per month left over in disposable income.

There is a graduated scale of charges for homemaker services. People with higher incomes pay more. There are no charges for people with the lowest incomes. On balance, the province collects about 3 to 5 percent of the total cost of homemaker programs from individual fees.

There is a $4 maximum daily charge for adult day-care centers, which covers meals, craft supplies, and so forth.

For Meals on Wheels, the individual is charged only for the cost of the food—typically about $3 for a hot, nutritious meal that would cost $6 to $10 in moderately priced restaurants. And there are no charges for home care nursing or for community physiotherapy programs.

The system employs several cost-control mechanisms, the most important being the very fact that it is a single-payer system. There also is control of supply. The province controls the number of beds involved and the number of homemaker hours provided. Centralized policy-making and planning enable the province to make decisions about what is required and where. The province controls the gatekeeping function, regulating who comes into the system and what mix of services each individual receives.

In addition to coordination of the long term care system with hospitals and with other parts of the Ministry of Health, there is coordination of long term care with other parts of government — for example, the Ministry of Attorney General works closely with the Ministry of Health in addressing issues of elder abuse.

Another cost-saving feature is that all residential care facilities have global budgets, similar to those in the hospital system. And there is a target ceiling on the number of hours each homemaker agency can provide, although the target can be exceeded in cases of exceptional community demand. Budgets and time allotments are worked out in terms of the needs of the communities involved.

Yet another cost-containment feature is the low administrative overhead cost, estimated at 1 to 1.5 percent of the total budget.

The overall system, then, draws its strength from several different concepts. It is a single-payer system. There is coordinated planning and policy-making. It is affordable to clients. There is a high level of consumer satisfaction. The case management approach allows control of gatekeeping. Accessibility is good.

The integrated nature of the program also allows for trade-offs. For example, if we want to manage the supply of beds and restrict the growth in the number of beds available in a particular area, we can shift more resources to the community care side and still remain within the overall balance of care and costs we have decided on.

The concept of choice is fundamental to the system. And, because the recipient of care — not the provider of care — is central to the whole program, the individual and the family are heavily involved in choosing the services appropriate to their needs.

Although overall control is at the provincial level, there is a fair amount of local flexibility. Within the basic system, one community may offer quite a different mix of services than another. For example, a community with a relatively younger and healthy elderly population may focus on programs such as supportive housing or adult day care, while another community might need a larger proportion of chronic care beds.

Weaknesses in the British Columbia system are those inherent in long term care systems everywhere.

One problem has been recruitment and retention in the home care support services industry. The industry suffers from high employee turnover rates, often on the order of 50 percent a year. But recent significant wage increases may help address this issue.

More geriatric specialists are needed, and other professionals should develop a better basic knowledge of geriatrics. A better level of awareness of aging issues in general is needed. The medical community must become more involved in care of the elderly. Some physicians are reasonably involved in care of the elderly, but others are hardly involved at all.

British Columbia needs to link the funding of its long term care system more closely with the quality of that care. The system now is primarily funded by a global grant. Even to the extent that the quality of service can be measured, there is little relationship between the level of quality and the level of funding.

But in considering the strengths and weaknesses of the Canadian long term care system, U.S. policy makers might do well to focus on how difficult it is to measure the success of any long term care system in isolation from the other elements of the health care system of which it is a part, such as hospitals and other acute care facilities. Can the success of one part of the system be measured as if it were independent of the rest? Or do the parts of the system have to be looked at as a total package of interconnecting government programs? Obviously, decisions in areas such as social housing or financial policy have dramatic effects on long term care of the elderly.

Whatever its shortcomings, as the Canadian long term care system evolves, the concept of an integrated delivery system for acute and long term care offers a society an enhanced opportunity for making sound decisions on how best to meet the needs of its citizens at an affordable cost.

In Canada, these decisions are made in partnership among government, provider, and individual. From our perspective, our health systems seem less adversarial and more cooperative than those of the United States. Perhaps that's just the nature of the Canadian people.

CHAPTER 8

Understanding the Health Care System That Works

Orvill Adams

Canada does not have nationalized health care. Canada has nationalized health insurance.

An appreciation of that often-blurred, but crucial, distinction is essential to understanding why the Canadian health care system — in reality as opposed to perception — is more like the U.S. system than it is like the "socialized medicine" systems of Europe and elsewhere.

It also explains why the myths that high-technology medicine is "rationed" in Canada and that its doctors quickly reach their income ceiling and spend the rest of the year basking on the beaches of Florida are just that — myths.

In fact, the way hospitals and doctors deal with health insurance in Canada is not fundamentally different from the way hospitals and doctors deal with U.S. insurance companies. The big difference in Canada is that the insurance "company" generally is the provincial government.

There is a continual tug over the dollar between Canadian health providers and insurers — just as there is a continual tug over the dollar in the United States between health providers and insurers.

The key difference is that, in Canada, the insurance company is owned, not by profit-minded shareholders, but by the

113

taxpayers—the same people who benefit from "free" medical care and are constantly balancing their desire for more and better service against their collective ability to pay for it.

It is this public ownership of the health insurance system—and the public debate underlying major policy decisions—that enables Canadians to enjoy health care comparable to, or better than, their U.S. neighbors, and at significantly lower cost.

The Canadian system is based on the core belief that access to health care—including nonmedical extended care at home or in a nursing home—should not be based on a person's ability to pay.

With that philosophical question settled, government leaders and health professionals can concentrate on improving the system—by introducing new technology at a pace that endangers neither the health nor the pocketbooks of the people, for example, and by devoting enough pennies to prevention to save substantial dollars on cures.

By a variety of mechanisms, mostly financial, government seeks to influence the ways health care is delivered, while those who deliver it—primarily hospital administrators and physicians—continue to assert their professional independence.

The result of this conflict seems to have been beneficial. Canadians get a quality of care most describe as good or excellent, physicians express satisfaction with their working conditions, and the costs are not excessive.

The Canadian health care system developed over many years, and its history is rooted in the political structure of the country.

Canada is a federation of provinces with a division of powers broadly similar to that of the United States. In the Constitution of 1867, health care was not specifically mentioned (except for marine hospitals and the care of Indians), but it has been decided that it lies within provincial jurisdiction.

Accordingly, early attempts at health care were largely local. The first decades of this century witnessed a variety of voluntary efforts at prepayment (or partial prepayment) for hospital and medical services. Friendly societies, mining companies, and railway union contracts were involved. In Saskatchewan and Alberta, for example, municipal medical and hospital programs were established, and in British Columbia, an attempt was made to introduce a provincewide program between 1935 and 1937. In 1947, Saskatchewan established a universal hospital program. British Columbia followed suit in 1949, and Alberta introduced its own plan in 1950.

By the early 1960s, many of the provinces had the elements of a health care system in place. For instance, Ontario, the most industrialized province, mandated hospital and medical care insurance for medium and large employee groups.

Although Canada's Parliament has long asserted complete control over the government process, there remains a gray area between legislative power and spending power. The Canadian federal government has used this imprecision to intrude into matters that are constitutionally within provincial jurisdiction, notably health care. By offering funds to the provincial government, under conditions laid out by legislation at the federal level, Parliament was able to influence and at times coerce the provinces into following its health care policies. Thus, in 1948, the federal government provided grants to the provinces for hospital construction and other public health initiatives. In 1958, the federal government provided payments for hospital care amounting to 25 percent of the provincial per-person spending plus 25 percent of national per-person spending.

The last major step came within the 1966 Medical Care Act, under which the federal government offered, in effect, to pay half the costs of medical care—50 percent of the national per-person expenditures multiplied by the number of insured persons in each province.

The provinces reacted in various ways. Some took the money. The Ontario premier angrily refused, accusing the federal government of using its spending power to reshape the Canadian Constitution. But with half of all federal revenue coming from Ontario, it made no sense for Ontario to refuse the federal largesse while still paying half the cost of the whole program. The province eventually fell into line, as did all the others.

The federal commitment to hospital and medical care funding was open ended, and as costs went up, this became a

concern to the federal treasury. In 1977, the payment formula
was changed to a block funding arrangement. Federal contributions were calculated from a base year (1975–76) and esca-
lated according to the growth of the gross national product
(GNP). This meant any province that could administer its health
care spending more efficiently would reap direct financial benefits.

The 1966 act required that, to receive the grants, provincial programs had to include five elements — public administration, comprehensiveness, universality, portability, and accessibility. The criteria were intended to ensure that Canadians
would be eligible for health care service without financial im-
pediment anywhere they went in Canada. The health services
were to be comprehensive in scope for medically necessary services, universal to all, and administered by a nonprofit public
agency. These criteria form the foundation for the national
character of the Canadian system. Canadians in the most economically disadvantaged province can be assured of access to
levels of care comparable to the care available in the more ad-
vantaged areas.

However, by the mid 1980s, there were complaints that
these criteria were not being satisfied. Critics of the system were
pointing to the numerous user charges that provincial governments were allowing to creep into the health care system. In
some provinces, hospitals were being allowed to impose daily
charges on patients. These charges were only a small part of
the total cost of each patient's hospital stay, but it was argued
that they were a barrier to access for proper health care for those
sickest and least able to pay. Even more serious, physicians were
allowed to increase their incomes by billing patients directly for
small amounts, in addition to billing the provincial paying
agency. This, too, was viewed as a barrier to appropriate health
care for those most vulnerable.

In 1984, the federal government introduced the Canada
Health Act, under which payments to provincial governments
were reduced by the amount estimated to be paid privately to
physicians for insured services. This had the effect of eliminating user charges and direct supplementary billing by physicians.

Now, only a relative handful of Canadians ever see a doctor bill. A very small number of physicians across the country insist on sending bills to their patients, who can then send the bills on to the provincial paying authority for reimbursement. In Quebec, however, if a physician practices outside of the plan, the patient is billed by and pays the physician directly but is not reimbursed by the government.

Drug costs and dental care were not covered by the 1966 federal plan, though in most provinces, some assistance with the cost of these services is provided. Most provinces pay the cost for the over-sixty-five age group and low-income residents. Other citizens have access to a variety of private plans, some negotiated as employee benefits.

Although the Canadian medical insurance system does not universally insure all long term care from the federal level, the national government started a block funding program in 1977 in which grants for extended care services are made to each province. The initial amount in 1977–78 was $20 for each person living in the province, escalated according to the growth of GNP. The development of long term care has not been even across the country. Provinces were given flexibility within the Canada Health Act to insure different long term care related services to different levels.

That has led to wide differences among the provinces, and many innovative models are being developed.

In many respects, the fundamental approach taken in Quebec of carefully assessing the needs of each individual is typical of the way long term care is handled throughout Canada.

Quebec Deputy Health Minister Duc Vu points out that the primary focus in Quebec is to enable an elderly person to remain in his or her own home as long as possible and to promote functional self-sufficiency. Institutionalization is prevented or delayed as long as practical.

Acute care hospitals in Quebec have specialized geriatric services available for those whose needs cannot be met at home but who do not require long term custodial care.

The third tier of care provides long term care in institutions for elderly people with severe functional disabilities or cognitive disorders. Nearly 43,000, or about 7 percent, of Quebec's

650,000 over sixty-five population are in long term care facilities. Most of them are women over the age of seventy-five.

Manitoba, for example, has found ways to provide a high level of home care assistance, perhaps thirty hours a week, at relatively low expense to the government by careful scheduling and an innovative approach to deciding how much is enough help for a particular individual.

Personal care attendants within the Manitoba system might be able to care for as many as seven people who are extremely disabled and get in and out to see those people at their homes during the day through careful scheduling. These care providers work directly for the province in Manitoba, but similar arrangements are worked out with private agencies in other provinces.

In other words, agencies don't have to set arbitrary four-hour minimums in order to send a home assistant to a particular location, or even two-hour minimums. Manitoba takes the stance that sometimes a person who is considered very disabled can nonetheless be left alone if they can call for and get help quickly if needed.

There are waiting lists for some Canadian nursing homes, but that does not mean people on the list are not getting appropriate care. Because the provincial systems provide for a continuum of care from home assistance to institutionalization, the person on a "waiting list" is merely waiting to move to another level of care. For example, if the person cannot stay at home and there is no room in the nursing home of his or her choice, this person might be kept in the long term care section of an acute care hospital for a few days or weeks until something opens up.

It's not as though the person were "languishing" without proper care.

A widely expressed concern is that people will abuse the opportunity to have home assistance — meals delivered, or house cleaning — by trying to obtain care beyond what they need. It's sometimes called the *woodwork effect* — people coming out of the woodwork to claim a need for a newly offered service such as home care.

But British Columbia's former Continuing Care Executive Director Paul Pallan says "our experience hasn't borne that out" in British Columbia. Speaking at a forum in Washington, D.C., Pallan explained, "Our view is that individuals choose to come in contact with the care system only when things have broken down, when things have happened to the point where they can't manage on their own. The other part of that is you have a managed system with checks and balances in terms of things like budgets, things like the number of hours and so forth. Inherently if you have a system which also has caps on spending there's going to be an internal distribution that means that those individuals who need the care the most are the ones that get the most care."[1]

At the same forum, Rosalie Kane called it "fascinating" that the woodwork effect is such a common concept in the United States and not in Canada.

"When we went in to study in Canada, basically with the woodwork effect in mind, we wanted to see how it had worked in British Columbia," she said.

"It looked as though — after an initial testing period, when a benefit was suddenly made available and obviously new people had to come on line — it just sort of settled down. You can really project the proportion of the population that need long term care. It's about 15 percent of the population over sixty-five, and you can work toward it.

"It doesn't seem to me that any province has experienced an unusual groundswell of people wanting services at home that were unreasonable."[2]

Physicians in Canada are for the most part individual entrepreneurs with the freedom to set up practice where they choose, subject to satisfying normal provincial licensing requirements. As consumers become more informed, physicians are challenged to be more responsive to their concerns. Similarly, as governments become more concerned with increasing health care costs, physicians are required to be accountable for their resource use, by placing greater emphasis on the quality and effectiveness of their treatment. Although there is an increasing movement to examine and use different remuneration and organizational methods to deliver health care services, physicians retain their autonomy to make professional decisions concerning the clinical care and management of their patients.

Just as U.S. physicians can take vacations whenever they want to, Canadian doctors also work for themselves and run their practices as they please, including scheduling their own hours and vacation times.

Some critics of the Canadian system, albeit usually those with limited experience with how it actually works, raise horror stories about Canadian doctors trying frantically to see as many patients as possible during the first months of the year until they have reached their income cap and then taking off for a sunny climate for months at a time.

The truth is, that just doesn't happen. For one thing, it would be as shortsighted for a Canadian doctor to run his or her practice that way — it simply wouldn't be good "business" — as it would be for a U.S. doctor to take a similar cavalier attitude. It would be a public relations disaster, and other physicians simply wouldn't stand for one of their colleagues operating this way. Peer review is a big factor in the Canadian system, with the medical associations keeping a close eye on how doctors operate under the system.

For another thing — even in the few provinces that cap doctor incomes — few Canadian doctors actually reach their caps. They are set in the first place, in negotiations between the medical associations and the governments, with an eye to projecting the level of service that will be needed during the coming year.

If the projections for a particular year are off target, the provinces employ a variety of mechanisms to take care of them in setting budgets for the following year. Doctors keep seeing patients even if they have reached their cap, keep submitting bills, and keep getting paid, although perhaps at a lower rate. In instances where a number have reached their ceiling and the government digs in against continuing payments at the 100 percent rate, the public debate may get quite noisy as the doctors position themselves for hard bargaining in hopes of setting higher limits for the coming year. They may even threaten to deliver only emergency or essential services for a while. These situations are widely covered in the media when they develop. But they don't arbitrarily close up shop and go to Florida. The media outcry alone probably would be enough to head off that kind of action.

On a more substantive level, however, the ethics of the Canadian medical profession simply doesn't allow this to happen. Canadian doctors are no less committed to the idea that their patients' welfare comes first than are their counterparts in the United States.

So there is some pulling and tugging when the money gets tight, but it all gets worked out.

Approaches designed to control utilization of physician services differ across the country. A series of measures have been negotiated with the medical profession. Both the government and the medical profession agree it is important to minimize unnecessary use of the system while ensuring that resources are available for necessary care. The 1989 agreement between the Alberta Medical Association and the government set caps for payments to physicians. As part of the monetary agreement, a "base increase" in utilization was also negotiated. The base was set at 1.5 percent to reflect increases that would be associated with demographic changes. The ministry agreed to full responsibility for the 1.5 percent increase. The medical profession agreed to be responsible for one-third of the increases above the initial 1.5 percent, by which physicians billing the plan would incur a corresponding prorated decrease in fees.

A memorandum of agreement between the Ontario government and the Ontario Medical Association also established income caps. The levels apply to gross fee-for-service billings to the Ontario Health Insurance Plan. In fiscal year 1991–92, there were two caps, $400,000 and $450,000. Physicians reaching the $400,000 cap in the fiscal year were paid at two-thirds the normal rate for fees above $400,000. Physicians reaching the cap of $450,000 were paid at a rate of one-third the normal billing rate over the cap. The caps — as generous as they may seem — do not apply to physicians in underserviced areas or to designated geographical or specialty areas. Some few physicians in the province expressed dissatisfaction with the cap; nevertheless, the profession overwhelmingly accepted the negotiated agreement.

By and large, utilization agreements negotiated between the provinces and the providers of care are not often significantly exceeded. Even when they are exceeded, what generally happens is that—in the next negotiations period—the utilization experience is discussed and the new agreement may be adjusted to reflect such factors as increased population growth, mix in population growth, new technology acquisition, change in disease patterns, epidemics, and so forth. The physicians may be asked to return a portion of earnings considered outside of the negotiated agreement.

Governments and provincial medical organizations are now actively working together to better understand the factors that contribute to increased use of the medical system. Both parties also are working together to develop and implement systems of clinical guidelines for practice.

Although at times there are conflicts between organized medicine and the governments, physicians are on the whole committed to the system.

If there were serious dissatisfaction with the system, one would expect a large number of physicians to choose to move to the United States because of its proximity and the opportunity to earn higher specialty incomes. This has not happened. In 1982, for example, emigrants amounted to 1.1 percent of the practicing physician pool. Since 1987, the figures have been less than 1 percent.[3]

Medicine also remains an attractive career for young Canadians. According to the Association of Canadian Medical Colleges, the number of applicants for each medical school position is between four and five. The corresponding measure for the United States is approximately 1.7.

Stevenson, Vayda, and Williams of York University and the University of Toronto conducted a national survey of Canadian physicians between November 1986 and May 1987. Sixty-one percent of respondents said they were satisfied or very satisfied in the practice of medicine at the present time, while only 24 percent were dissatisfied or very dissatisfied. More than half the physicians surveyed were satisfied with their own working conditions, their ability to keep up their professional knowledge, and their access to support staff and equipment. On the other hand, only 49 percent were satisfied or very satisfied with their financial security, despite their status as Canada's highest-paid profession.[4]

Hospitals are funded largely through global budgets, which finance approximately 90 percent of the operating cost of hospitals, with the government paying two-thirds of capital costs. This allows the government to work with the hospitals and the providers to rationalize investment in bed capacity and medical technology acquisition.

Until recently, hospitals that incurred deficits applied to the government for additional financing and for the most part received it. This led to cases of chronic deficit financing, because hospitals were not forced to be more cost effective. Governments across the country are now insisting that they will not provide additional funds for deficit financing unless the hospitals can demonstrate that there are no organizational or management strategies that can be used to realize savings while *not* jeopardizing the quality of patient care.

Hospitals have therefore adopted strategies intended to streamline their operations through improved management information systems and better allocation of physical and human resources. Some hospitals have closed beds and consolidated service delivery during slower periods of demand. Greater use of ambulatory care services, which is better for the patients — and saves money — also is being promoted.

If the hospitals, despite all their efforts, are unable to stay within budget and ensure quality care, governments provide additional financing. The Health Ministry may, however, require the hospitals to prepare detailed reports about their operations and conduct studies that will help them be more effective and efficient in the future. In a few cases of poor management, provincial governments have imposed their own manager until performance improves.

There are no rigid expenditure caps within the Canadian

health care system. Instead, there are mechanisms that set de facto expenditure targets to encourage better management and use of resources. The experience has always been that if medical need is demonstrated, the financing will be available. The policies and strategies of global budgeting and utilization management are intended to encourage greater emphasis on the provision of effective, necessary health care.

All of these decisions at the provincial level take place within the context of rigid federal mandates that *all* medically necessary treatment be provided, *not* that the province may limit care on grounds of cost-effectiveness.

The Canadian health care system delivers services to the whole population at relatively lower costs than the United States. This difference is largely due to our single-payer system in each province, allowing for relatively low administrative costs, approximately $21 per capita. A 1991 U.S. General Accounting Office report on Canadian health insurance acknowledges that costs associated with marketing competitive health insurance policies, billing for and collecting premiums, and evaluating insurance risks can be significantly reduced by using a universal publicly financed single-payer system. The report points out that Canada's per capita spending on health insurance administration was only one-fifth that of the United States in 1987.[5]

In 1989, Canada spent the equivalent of U.S. $1,739 per capita for health care, while the United States spent $2,354, a difference of $615 per person. Estimates for 1990 placed U.S. per capita spending at $2,425, compared to $1,888 in Canada, again in U.S. dollars.[6]

The growth in nominal per capita health spending has shown similar trends in both countries. In a 1989 article for *Health Affairs,* Schieber and Poullier reported that for the period 1980–1987, the annual growth rates were 9.9 and 9.4 percent respectively for Canada and the United States. Similarly, *real* annual per capita health expenditure for 1980–1987 grew at 1.5 percent in Canada and 1.7 percent in the United States.[7]

Comparisons between the U.S. and Canadian systems often focus on the similarity of health care costs as a share of national income in the two countries in 1971 (7.6 percent in the United States and 7.4 percent in Canada) and on the differences that are observed beginning in 1975 (see Table 8.1). The health care system in Canada was relatively stable throughout the 1970s. The share of the GNP devoted to the health care sector rose sharply during the recession of 1982 in both countries.

Table 8.1. Health Care Expenditures as a Percentage of Gross National Product, Canada and the United States, Selected Years 1960–1990.

Year	Health Expenditure as a Percent of GNP	
	Canada	United States
1960	5.6	5.3
1965	6.2	6.0
1970	7.3	7.5
1975	7.5	8.6
1980	7.5	9.5
1981	7.7	9.7
1982	8.5	10.5
1983	8.8	10.5
1984	8.7	10.4
1985	8.6	10.6
1987	9.0	11.0
1989	8.9	11.6
1990	9.2	12.0

Source: Data from Health and Welfare Canada, *National Health Expenditures, 1970–1982* and *1975–1985;* Health and Welfare Canada, 1984, 1987, 1989, 1990 (yearly reports).

The Canadian health care system is financed through a mix of public and private funds. In 1988, the federal government contributed 30 percent, the provincial governments 42 percent, and the private sector 25 percent of all money spent on health care. Local government and workers' compensation accounted for the remainder. During the 1970s, nongovernmental health care spending in Canada fell from 30 percent of the total at the beginning of the decade to a low of 23 percent in 1975, only to rise to 25 percent in 1979 and 1980.[8]

Among countries in the Organization for Economic Cooperation and Development (OECD), the share of total health expenditures borne by the public sector averaged 76 percent. The public sector share in Canada in 1987 was approximately 74 percent. The corresponding share in the United States was 41 percent.

Provincial government contributions are funded primarily through general revenue. Quebec and Manitoba supplement general revenue with a payroll tax on employers of 3.2175 percent and 2.25 percent, respectively. In 1989, Ontario announced that it would move from a combination of general revenue and premiums to an employer health levy (EHL). Companies reporting total annual gross wages, salaries, and other remuneration in excess of $400,000 contribute 1.95 percent of their payroll, while companies reporting less than $200,000 pay 0.98 percent, with companies between these levels paying on a graduated scale.

Before 1989, Ontario financed its health care system with a combination of general revenue and premiums. These individual and family premiums were viewed by many as a "health care tax." This tax covered 16.2 percent of total health care spending for Ontario in 1985–86. Alberta and British Columbia continue to raise revenues in this manner. In addition, British Columbia levies an 8 percent health maintenance tax based on personal income tax.

Many analysts criticize this method as an unfair and inefficient way of financing the health care system. A recent unpublished report of the National Council of Welfare examines premiums in Alberta and British Columbia. The analysis found that despite premium subsidies, the premiums do not in any way take a person's ability to pay into consideration. "The one-earner couple with two children and taxable income of $22,000 paid about 2 percent of taxable income in Medicare premiums in 1989–1990. The family with taxable income of $100,000 paid less than ½ of 1 percent."[9]

This is a serious criticism, especially because the question of equity impacts on health outcomes. The relationship between income and health status has received increased attention in the past few years. Wilkins and Adams, writing in *Illusions of Necessity: Evading Responsibility for Choice in Health Care,* found that "healthfulness of life was directly related to income whether the measure was overall life expectancy, disability-free life or quality-adjusted life expectancy."[10]

About 40 cents of the Canadian health care dollar goes to hospitals. In 1986, there were 171,936 beds in operation, representing 6.72 beds per 1,000 population. Of the total, 112,275 beds were designated short-term care units and 59,661 long term care units. The number of short-term beds per 1,000 population fell from 5.25 in 1975 to 4.39 in 1986. In contrast, long term care beds per 1,000 population increased from 1.66 in 1975 to 2.33 in 1986.

The share of health dollars devoted to hospitals decreased from 44 percent to 39 percent between 1975 and 1988. Expenditures for other institutions grew from 10 percent in 1975 to 11 percent in 1978 and averaged more than 11 percent during the period 1978–1983. In the last three years for which data are available, the proportion has been stable at 10 percent. The change reflects policies by governments to encourage greater use of ambulatory settings.

Physicians' services are the second largest component of health care expenditures. They remained very stable during the 1980s, averaging 16 percent between 1978 and 1988. Dentists' services average around 5 percent.

The share of spending for prescribed and nonprescribed drugs increased from 9 percent in 1975 to 12 percent in 1988.

About 65 percent of Canadians have private health insurance for medication, and an additional 20 percent are covered by provincial drug plans. Over the years, these provincial plans have increased the proportion of prescription drugs for which they pay. Ontario now covers more than 40 percent of all prescriptions.

Attempts to control rising pharmaceutical costs have included establishment of lists of drugs for which the province will pay. Strategies such as substitution of lower-cost drugs and greater emphasis on the effectiveness of particular drug treatments are being pursued.

Capital construction, repair, and acquisitions have consumed a declining share of total expenditures as provincial governments have become much more stringent in their allocation of capital budgets. This has resulted in a greater reliance on funds from the private sector through philanthropy. Hospitals

also are becoming more involved in marketing ventures in an
effort to increase their capital funds.

One of the areas in which there has been rapid growth
in dollar terms is home care. However, this area still remains
a very small part of total health care expenditures, making up
approximately 1 percent. Over the past ten years, provincial
governments "have been actively developing home and early discharge programs, signalling a commitment to more, and less
costly, types of care," according to Earl J. Gallant, chair of the
Nova Scotia Royal Commission on Health Care.[11]

The Canadian health care system is organized and managed slightly differently in each province. This is partially re-
flected in the differences in per capita spending across the country. The per capita spending ranges from a high of $1,985 in
Ontario to a low of $1,473 in Newfoundland. The share of gross
domestic product (GDP) consumed by the health care sector
in 1987 varied across the provinces, from a high of slightly over
12 percent in relatively poor Prince Edward Island to a low of
slightly under 7 percent in relatively rich Alberta.

Health expenditures consume between 25 and 34 percent
of provincial government expenditures. Ontario spent approximately $12.5 billion in 1989 and an estimated $13.6 billion in
1990. Ontario health care expenditures in 1990 were $15.3 bil-
lion and were estimated to have reached $17.2 billion in 1991,
accounting for 34 percent of the province's government expenditures.

Hospital bed use also varies across the provinces. In 1986,
the number of beds per 1,000 population ranged from a high
of 7.9 in Quebec to a low of 5.5 in Ontario. These differences
reflect the degree of development of ambulatory care and home
care programs. Canadian hospitals for the most part have relatively high occupancy rates, and these rates rose during the 1970s
and 1980s. The national average was 84 percent in 1986.

The average length of stay in inpatient institutions was
13.2 days in 1987. Since 1981, the Canadian average length
of stay has fluctuated between 13.1 and 13.6 days. This is strikingly longer than south of the border. In 1986 (the last year for
which data are available) the average length of stay in the United

States was 9.6 days, four days less than the comparable Canadian figure. Admission rates in Canada also are higher than rates in the United States, as are occupancy rates.

George J. Schieber, director of the Office of Research for the U.S. Health Care Financing Administration, said in a 1988 presentation before Congress' Joint Economic Subcommittee on Education and Health that "although average length of stay per admission is less in the United States, expenditures per day and per admission are substantially higher than those in other countries." He offered three possible reasons: (1) that the intensity of services per day and per stay is higher in the United States, (2) that the amenity levels are higher, and (3) that there is inefficiency and waste in the U.S. system. Schieber cautions, however, that until we have better measures of outcome, it is difficult to make judgments about the relative performance of American hospitals.[12]

One thing that is clear is that consumers of health care in Canada live longer than consumers of health care in the United States. But even within Canada, there are significant variations in life expectancy from province to province. In 1985–1987 (the last years for which data are available), the life expectancy at birth for males varied from a high of 74.1 years in British Columbia to a low of 72.0 years in Quebec. The Canadian average for males was 73.0 years. The national average for females was 79.7 years. Saskatchewan's women fared best with a life expectancy of 80.5 years, and Nova Scotia's women had the lowest life expectancy at 79.2 years.

Life expectancy varies not only by province but also by income, although the life expectancy gap among income groups has narrowed since the Canadian health care system came into being. In 1971, there was a difference in life expectancy of 2.8 years between the poorest and richest groups. This had fallen to 1.8 years by 1986.[13] Although improvement in health status depends on more than health care services, improvements in access to health care services for the disadvantaged cannot be ignored as a contributing factor.

In the fifteen years between 1971 and 1986, life expectancy at birth increased for all income groups, but it was middle-

income men and women who experienced the largest increase
in life expectancy at birth, and the gap between middle-income
Canadians and rich Canadians closed dramatically.

It is hard to compare health care utilization from country to country because there are different definitions, different
measurement methods, and varied patterns of practice. One indicator of physician use is the number of physician-patient contacts. By this measure, Canadians clearly get more attention
from doctors than do their neighbors to the south. Simone San-
dier, working with the OECD in 1989 while on sabbatical from
the Centre de Recherche d'Etude et de Documentation en Econ-
omie de la Santé, found that in 1985 Canada had 7.2 physician
contacts per person, compared to 5.4 in the United States. Her
results also indicated that, in countries where a referral from
a general practitioner is not necessary, the use of specialists' services is greater. In Canada, a referral from a general practitioner is not necessary, but the specialist is paid more for a consultation done as the result of a referral. While Canadians have
more contacts with physicians as a whole, they have significantly
fewer with specialists: 2.5 annually per person, as compared to
3.7 in the United States.

Surgical utilization rates for coronary bypass and angiography are dramatically greater in the United States. This is not
the case for pacemaker implants, prostatectomy, and total hip
replacements, which are more common in Canada, nor for
cholecystectomy, which is minimally more common in the United
States. The differences in utilization have not resulted in poorer
health for Canadians. In fact, the Canadian health care system
has performed at least as well as the U.S. system and arguably
far better in terms of ensuring a comparable degree of health
status of the population served. The OECD reports demonstra-
bly better life expectancy figures for Canada as compared to
the United States for both males and females. In 1984, the life
expectancy at birth for Canadian males was 73.0 years, versus
71.1 for American males. For females, the life expectancy at
birth in 1984 was 79.8 years in Canada and 78.3 in the United
States. Despite the disparity between blacks and whites in the
U.S., life expectancy for *whites* in the United States in 1984

Table 8.2. Comparative Utilization of Selected
Surgical Procedures, Procedures per 10,000 Population, 1987.

Procedure	Procedures per 10,000 Population	
	Canada	United States
Coronary bypass	6.6	13.7
Angiography	33.1	41.0
Pacemaker implants	3.2	2.8
Prostatectomy	22.2	17.0
Cholecystectomy	21.2	22.2
Total hip replacement	10.8	8.6
Procedure	Procedures per 10,000 Population Aged 65+	
	Canada	United States
Coronary bypass	24.0	50.9
Angiography	96.1	122.3
Pacemaker implants	16.4	16.8
Prostatectomy	136.1	106.9
Cholecystectomy	45.7	57.3
Total hip replacement	64.5	53.3

Source: "Cost Implications, Fiscal Alternatives and Rationing the Level of Care," unpublished manuscript, Department of Health, British Columbia, 1990.

was 71.8 years for males and 78.7 years for females — still lower than the Canadian figures for *all races*. In terms of age-standardized death rates per 100,000, Canada had 761.8 deaths in 1984, while the available figure for the United States in 1983 was 915.8 per 100,000 population.

OECD reports that the infant mortality rate in Canada in 1986 was 8.0 deaths per 1,000 live births, while in the United States, the corresponding figure was 10. The infant mortality rate for *whites* in the United States was 9.4 deaths per 1,000 live births, dramatically higher than rates for *all races* in Canada.

In this context, it is worthwhile to explore the Canadian approach to medical technology.

One of the fundamental reasons costs are lower in Canada is the way the growth of new, expensive, and sometimes untested (and potentially dangerous) technology is controlled through the requirement that all major technology services be delivered in hospitals and institutions. In order for an institution to add a new service, such as a new MRI scanner, a lithotripter, or a cardiac surgical unit, it must go to government to get approval for increased operating budgets to begin the service.

This control, however, is not meant to compromise the quality of care being offered and in practice seldom has that effect. Despite the occasional anecdote that gets wildly overblown in the media, the Canadian approach to measured introduction of new technology does not amount to rationing of health care. There are lapses, as there will be in any system, but these oversights are self-correcting because of the way the system is designed and because of the high level of public attention devoted to such incidents.

Greg Stoddart and David Feeny, health economists at the Centre for Health Economics and Policy Analysis, suggest that the underlying policies governing health care technology in Canada are appropriate diffusion and appropriate utilization. Provincial governments strive with some success, especially with the "big-ticket items," to ensure appropriate diffusion through research and evaluation before dissemination and use in selected clinical settings. They argue that "appropriate diffusion would ensure that major new technologies are provided in amounts that correspond to health care needs (constrained by society's ability and willingness to pay) and that such technologies are appropriately located within a jurisdiction." They also define appropriate utilization as the "application of technology to cases and conditions where its use is known to be effective."[14]

The introduction and diffusion of the more expensive medical technologies are controlled by provincial governments. The appropriate number, use, and assessment of both diagnostic and therapeutic technologies and the rising cost of such technologies are increasingly debated within the Canadian health care system. Pranlal Manga, an economist and commentator on ethics and resource allocation, makes the following six observations about medicine, technology, and costs.[15]

1. The diffusion of new technologies is frequently too rapid and occurs without adequate evaluation and assessment.

2. While it appears that medical technology has contributed to rising health care costs and expenditures, it is not clear nor easy to specify which technology is the problem, and the scale to which specific technologies are a problem.

3. Some medical technologies in widespread use have been retrospectively proven to be ineffective and sometimes harmful.

4. One of the main reasons that medical technology engenders higher health care costs is its excessive and inappropriate use by the professions in the various health care delivery systems. This overuse applies to both diagnostic and therapeutic technologies.

5. Technologies are introduced and diffused even when the marginal benefits (of improved health) are relatively small and uncertain relative to large and certain marginal costs.

6. Technological approaches to disease and disability are sought without considering, and sometimes in spite of, known and cost-effective therapies. Disease prevention and health promotion alternatives have similarly been ignored or overlooked.

Unlike in the United States, the diffusion of medical technology in Canada is also governed by the basic goal of the Canadian health care system — equity of distribution of services across Canada.

In a system of rationing, equity would mean that medically necessary services would be denied equitably to patients. That is not the goal of any province's health care system; the Canadian federal government requires that provinces ensure that medically necessary services are denied to nobody. Are there shortfalls, despite the guarantees of the Canada Health Act? Of course. But they are not part of the system. Whenever they occur, there is an effort to overcome them through better management or increased spending.

Shortfalls in the availability of certain high-tech medical services are not endemic. By intent, and in practice, the Canadian system seeks to avoid shortfalls and to cure them when — as a result of bad planning or other circumstances — they do appear.

Through political pressures and pressures originating in the media, both the general public and physicians and other providers have a significant impact on the diffusion of medical technology in Canada. The Canadian health care system is highly politicized. The media provides regular coverage, and health care is always a key political issue.

Provider groups have in fact begun to assume some of the responsibility for the adoption and use of new medical technologies before the cost and benefits have been assessed. The Ontario Medical Association (OMA) took a brave step in addressing the difficult questions of cost, resource allocation, and ethics when it tackled the debate over the use of two thrombolytic agents in acute myocardial infarction: tissue-type plasminogen activator (tPA) and streptokinase. The cost of tPA is ten times that of streptokinase. The OMA reported that it "convened a meeting of a group of cardiologists and internists who were asked to produce recommendations for appropriate use of coronary thrombolytic agents, given due consideration to proven clinical indications and the need to avoid indiscriminate waste of scarce resources." Bolstered by the knowledge that the international cardiology community had recommended the continuing use of streptokinase, OMA distributed guidelines for the use of thrombolytic agents in March 1988.[16]

The flexibility of the Canadian system is demonstrated in the response from Ontario. The provincial government did not take account of the increased cost of tPA in its global budgets; nevertheless, hospitals that made special requests for funds to use tPA received them. The decision in this case was being made not by the government, but by individual hospital boards and administrators, most often with significant input from physicians.

There is an increasing movement within the Canadian system toward questioning the quality and health benefits derived from the use of new technologies. As a partial response, technology assessment programs have been established recently in Quebec, Ontario, and British Columbia. In addition, the federal government has established the Canadian Coordinating

Office for Health Technology Assessment. Its purpose is to provide information and a framework that can be used by policy makers, providers, and funding agencies in the dissemination and use of both new and old diagnostic and therapeutic technology. While emphasis is being placed on new technologies, the system is turning its attention to the need for continued and more vigorous evaluation of established technologies.

Canada's management of health care technology has resulted in differences in the availability of medical technologies in the system as compared to other countries. Dale Rublee, of the American Medical Association, undertook a study of the comparative availability of selected medical technologies in Canada, Germany, and the United States.

Rublee's figures refer only to the facilities for treatment, not the use made of them, their availability, or — as Rublee put it — "differing views of physicians and patients about the indications for procedures." His study showed that Canada had far fewer facilities for open-heart surgery, cardiac catheterization, radiation therapy, lithotripsy, and magnetic resonance imaging than the United States, and somewhat fewer organ transplant facilities. Rublee's study did not look at the intensity of use of the facilities in each country or at the implications of differences in intensity of use on the quality of care.[17]

Criticisms of the Canadian system based on differences in capacity fail to consider effectiveness, health outcomes, and access of the general population to health care services. It is worth repeating that although the United States has higher rates of use in a number of selected surgical areas, health status measures do not indicate that Canadians are less healthy than residents of the United States.

A report of the British Columbia Department of Health shows that in 1989, British Columbia had one magnetic resonance imaging facility per million persons, as compared to Rublee's 3.69 facilities per million people in the United States. On the other hand, the British Columbia report points out that another technological benchmark — the rate of kidney transplantation in British Columbia — is one of the highest in any jurisdiction in North America.

What seems clear is that differences in availability of technologies between Canadian provinces and American states reflect a range of causes. And while both oversupply and temporary shortages of certain technologies occur from time to time in one or another Canadian province, neither oversupply nor shortage is endemic to the Canadian health care system.

Rather, the Canadian system is particularly well equipped to respond to the need for change and improvement, for the very good reason that problems tend to rapidly become quite public — and responsibility rests squarely with the government to see that improvements are made.

Although the lower use of technology in Canada than in the United States may reflect problems of excessive caution in introducing new approaches in Canada, it may also reflect inadequate caution and overutilization in the United States. One way to absolutely avoid waiting lines for elective surgery is to build excess capacity into the system. The United States has de facto chosen that approach for some technologies.

There has been a great deal of U.S. media attention to waiting lines for elective surgery in Canada. (Just as shortages in U.S. cities in areas such as emergency room medicine have attracted attention.) There has not been the same amount of media attention to the question of whether excess capacity — in either country — has led to decreased quality in underutilized facilities or to an increase in unnecessary surgery, with the attendant increased risk to patients. There are, nonetheless, serious critics in both countries who worry that excess capacity is a significant threat to patient well-being.

As an example, Canada's rate for surgical obstetrical deliveries in 1989 was 20 percent, four times higher than the Netherlands, which records the lowest rate in the industrialized world. The corresponding figure for the United States is even higher, at 25 percent. The appropriateness of these levels in both Canada and the United States must be questioned.

Inappropriate use can lead to a reduction in health care quality. Dr. Hugh Scully, deputy head and professor of cardiovascular surgery at The Toronto Hospital, where twenty-three heart transplants were performed in 1991, argues that more than

80 percent of the 1,200 transplants done in the United States annually are performed in centers that do fewer than ten a year, "and that's not sufficient to maintain competence."[18]

It has long been established that surgical procedures such as coronary bypass have lower complication rates when performed in hospitals — and by surgeons — that do a substantial number. Similarly, diagnostic procedures such as mammography are more dependable when performed in higher-volume facilities.

One of the clear advantages of the relatively tight control Canadian provinces exercise over the dissemination of new technology is to concentrate it in a way that ensures high volume of usage in fewer centers. Similarly, slowing down dissemination of new technology can help avoid creating incentives for dangerous overuse of the technology.

But, in the constant weighing of the disadvantages of too-rapid dissemination of new technology against the disadvantages of too cautious dissemination, the Canadian health care system has one key advantage: the responsiveness of elected governments to public dissatisfaction with the way the system is working.

As an example, over the past few years, increases in waiting lists for cancer treatment and cardiovascular care have drawn much media attention.

In Ontario, the Ontario Cancer Institute (OCI), which operates the Princess Margaret Hospital and other hospitals in Toronto, was faced with a crisis brought on by an underestimation of the number of radiotherapy machines that would be needed as well as the number of technicians to operate them.

While additional machines were being obtained, an international recruitment drive for radiation technologists was conducted, resulting in an increase of ninety-five technologists by the fall of 1990. A training committee was put in place to examine the available programs and to make recommendations for expanded or new programs. As a short-term solution, patients were referred to other centers in and outside of the province.

The Ministry of Health in Ontario has increased its funding for cancer services by $300 million over four years and it has created the Ontario Cancer Control Agency, which will be responsible for ensuring a coordinated network of cancer services throughout the province.

Another high-profile pressure point within the Canadian health care system centers on increasing waiting times for cardiovascular services. Dr. David Naylor, a researcher at the University of Toronto, reported in the *Canadian Medical Association Journal* that in Ontario, "Waiting lists for elective coronary artery bypass surgery during 1988 ranged between two and 12 months in five of the nine hospitals with open heart surgery facilities and the three cardiac centers in Toronto had a combined waiting list of 848 patients as of January 1989."[19] The Ministry of Health responded quickly to the perceived crisis by taking the following initiatives:

- Increasing funding at a number of hospitals and cardiovascular treatment centers across the province.
- Forming a committee to investigate the quality of cardiac care at St. Michael's Hospital in Toronto, where there had been a much-publicized death of a patient awaiting elective surgery.
- Creating a network for adults and a parallel network for children to coordinate expanding cardiovascular services. The network links cardiovascular units across the province. Patient management teams were set up to list all cardiovascular patients awaiting surgery in a central regional registry to keep the queue of patients moving smoothly. A coordinator in each region informs doctors and patients of their status on the waiting lists; patients requiring urgent surgery that could not be performed locally, as well as patients awaiting elective surgery who wanted to shorten the wait for surgery, were referred to another region.

In April 1991, waiting times in Ontario were estimated to be no more than seven weeks on average, down from the high crisis levels in 1988.

The factors contributing to increasing pressures and waiting lists for cardiovascular services are complex. They include demographics, changing patterns of practice, service capacity, and the availability of appropriate human resources.

The much reported increase in cardiac surgical waiting lists in Vancouver in 1989 is often cited by American critics of Canada's health care system as a symptom of fundamental weakness in our system. In fact, it represents an instance of the flexibility of our system. The increase in waiting lists was caused in part by a hospital employees' strike and a shortage of critical care nurses and perfusionists, the technicians who operate heart-lung machines during operations. The pressure was not brought on by government cutbacks in funding, because allowances had been made for funding open-heart cases. (Funding is adjusted at the beginning of each year based on the disease patterns of the population, hospital capacity, and previous utilization.)

As a short-term measure, the British Columbia ministry arranged for some patients to have their surgery performed at hospitals in the United States, Seattle in particular. Given that the U.S. hospitals were operating at about 60 percent capacity, ministry officials were able to negotiate favorable terms. Capacity was in fact available in other hospitals in the province: patients could have been sent from Vancouver to Victoria instead of to Seattle.

In all, the total number of patients sent to Seattle was no more than 200 over two years, out of more than 5,000 open-heart surgeries performed in British Columbia in those years.

As in other countries, the Canadian health care system will face increasing pressures in the coming years, including demographic changes, growth in medical technology, growth in physician supply, and growth in the use of health care services.

The changing age distribution of the Canadian population is expected to lead to increases in the cost of provision of health care services. The proportion of the population over sixty-five in 1981 was just under 10 percent. This was expected to reach a little under 12 percent by 1991 and 17 percent by 2021. As the distribution of the population changes, the result may not only be a demand for more service, but also a demand for different services.

All provincial governments have expressed concern about the growth in physician supply and the associated cost. At the same time, they are faced with maldistribution by specialty and geography. The need to increase the supply of nurses and improve their working conditions and retention rates has also been identified as a priority area for governments.

Public and provider expectations continue to grow in the face of the need for provincial governments to be fiscally responsible in the management of their health care systems.

Governments have responded to these growing concerns by establishing provincial task forces and commissions with broad representation from consumers and providers. The mandates of these reviews have been to study and report on ways to improve their respective health care systems. Since 1983, all governments except that of Prince Edward Island have employed this device to examine their systems. Recommendations coming out of these commissions are similar in nature, addressing issues of financing and human resources organization and management, as well as more specific issues, such as service to targeted populations (for example, the disabled, rural residents, and native peoples).

The underlying theme of the reports to date can be said to be a desire to shift the system away from its preoccupation with the delivery of health care services to a broader perspective that increasingly considers the promotion of health and the prevention of disease. There is also a common theme of regionalization of services and decentralized management of resources. Provinces continue to experiment and make changes designed to improve their systems, under the continuing pressure of political reality: governments that allow health care to lag behind public expectations do not get reelected.

Canadians are generally satisfied but not complacent about their health care system. The Canadian system remains highly politicized, which is seen as both an advantage and a disadvantage. The disadvantage is that interest groups can easily elevate manageable difficulties to major crises through the media. The enormous advantage is the high degree of responsiveness of the system to the people who use it.

The Canadian health care system is undergoing a number of changes, adjusting to the different pressures it faces. Canadians remain committed to equitable provision of services to all, regardless of their ability to pay and based on medical indication. They continue to express extreme concern and even outrage if they perceive that the system may be threatened.

Many challenges face the Canadian system as governments seek efficiencies in difficult fiscal times. Policy analysts, researchers, and health care providers are promoting maintenance and improvement of quality, and the public is increasingly demanding greater accountability from government and from health care providers. These concerns are being answered by initiatives that provide the opportunity for communities to have a greater say in the way health care services are organized and delivered. Canadians will continue to reassess and modify their health care system in order to ensure that all Canadians have access to quality hospital and medical care services.

CHAPTER 9

Eleven Lessons from Canada's Health Care System

Ron Pollack

Jeffrey R. is eight years old. He plays soccer. He's a Cub Scout. Sometimes he fights with his brothers. He looks and sounds like a bright, healthy, happy kid.

That's how he seems, during the day. At night, things are very different.

Jeffrey has a birth defect in his brain stem, which causes him to stop breathing when he falls asleep. All night, every night, he must be hooked up to machines that monitor his blood-oxygen levels and keep him breathing, setting off alarms when his breathing stops. All night, every night, he is watched by a nurse who monitors the thousands of dollars' worth of high-tech machinery that crowds a corner of his bedroom.

Like any family hit by serious illness, Jeffrey's problem has been physically difficult and emotionally draining for the whole family. Illness is always a traumatic experience, anywhere in the world.

But because Jeffrey lives in the United States, his illness is not just physically and emotionally painful. It is also a financial catastrophe for his family. The current system of private health insurance has proved itself to be inadequate to the needs of middle-income families like his.

Anywhere in the world, when medical disaster strikes,

families are plunged into pain and worry and insecurity. But in the United States, that misery is all too often compounded by the fear that the cost of health care can bankrupt you. This critical failure of the current private insurance system is all too apparent to Jeffrey's family.

"We thought we had excellent health insurance. But Jeffrey spent most of his first nineteen months in the hospital," Sandy, Jeffrey's mother, relates. "By the time Jeffrey was eleven months old, his $100,000 lifetime policy limit was used up. The last time I checked, we owed them $600,000 from back bills, because there was a period of time from eleven months until he was about four years old where he had no insurance whatsoever, nor did we qualify for Medicaid."

The family already knows it will never be out of debt. Jeffrey's dad, Rick, is an electrician and Sandy is training to be a respiratory therapist. But they know their entire life's earnings will never equal Jeffrey's health care bills, and the interest that is piling up. And the family doesn't know what will happen to Jeffrey when he turns eighteen and his Medicaid assistance ends.

The family's story is not unusual. Medical bankruptcy is a nightmare facing more Americans every day. And, because of cost, many working- and middle-class American families don't get the care they need.

Sandy feels that the only reason Jeffrey received care, in the end, was that she fought for it tooth and nail. She fought for ongoing care even though charges sometimes reached $2,000 a day, and despite the fact that it took months for doctors to figure out what was wrong.

The fact that many Americans postpone care they need because they fear the costs is a symptom of a wider tragedy. America has sunk into a health care crisis.

The emergency touches every one of us. Working families discover that their private health insurance lets them down when serious illness strikes. There are higher and higher copayments. When people change jobs, they risk losing their insurance.

When an employer switches insurance companies, employees may lose their coverage. Some workers face long waiting periods before insurance benefits kick in; others find that their illnesses are classed as "preexisting conditions," which won't ever be covered.

Many workers simply can't afford protection for their family. The fact is that health care costs are skyrocketing. Health cost inflation now runs at more than twice the general rate of inflation. Between 1980 and 1990, health spending in the United States almost tripled; we expect it to more than double again by the end of the decade. Our health spending for 1990 was more than $2,425 for every man, woman, and child in the United States. And that will go up to $5,515 per year by the year 2000.

Even with these incredible levels of spending, we cannot afford to keep critical medical services operating, because we don't spend that money wisely. So in our big cities—Miami, Houston, Philadelphia, Washington, and others—hospital trauma centers are closing down because they can't afford to stay open. All of us, regardless of how well insured we may be, now face the threat of delays in getting emergency care in the event of an accident or heart attack.

Everyday health care also is endangered. The United States is falling behind other industrialized countries in the general health of our citizens. A host of studies bear this out. We Americans die younger—*years* younger than Canadians or Germans or Japanese. Americans suffer higher death rates from heart disease. Our children suffer alarming rates of preventable diseases such as measles, rubella, and whooping cough. Our babies suffer more from low birthweight than babies born in twenty-three other countries. The United States now ranks twentieth among nations in terms of the health of infants (as measured by infant mortality), when we should rank no. 1.[1]

Why is this happening in a country with resources second to none? Why does the United States have a health care system that forces middle-income parents to think twice before getting their prescriptions filled or taking their kids for a checkup?

Our health care system is in trouble because we are financing it the wrong way.

Increasingly, we are learning that we can't provide high-quality health care for a nation through an inflated, fragmented system that wastes billions of dollars each year on red tape, overcharges, and mismanagement.

Can we provide better care for our families? Can we ensure quality of care and still control its cost?

The evidence from Canada is that it *can* be done.

Canada, our closest neighbor and in many ways the country most like us, has an immensely successful health care system. Judging by health outcomes, it can be argued that Canada provides better care than we receive. Canadians live longer. Their babies are healthier. Their old folks are better looked after. They suffer lower death rates from preventable diseases such as heart disease. And they do all this while paying less for health care than we do. Because they organize it right, and we don't.

There are two reasons the lessons of the Canadian health care financing system can be so instructive to us.

First, as Robert Evans points out, our health care *delivery* systems are really quite similar.

Second, our fundamental beliefs are also much alike. The criteria by which the Canadians can measure their success are, after all, the same criteria that we as Americans use to measure our own system: availability of high-quality care, fairness, affordability, confidentiality of the doctor-patient relationship, and freedom of choice.

Taking a close look at Canada does not suggest it has the only successful health system in the industrialized world — there are many things to learn from the Germans, the Japanese, and others — or that we should adopt the Canadian system. We won't. We'll achieve distinctly American reform.

With Bill Clinton in the White House with a health reform mandate, the opportunity for comprehensive health care reform is greater than at any time in the past. And the single most important lesson we can learn from Canada is that it is *possible* to deliver high-quality health care to all the people of a great nation without breaking the bank.

Here, then, are eleven lessons we can draw by looking north for health.

Lesson 1: You Don't Always Get What You Pay For

The United States spends more than Canada for health care, but do Americans receive more?

Many variables make it hard to compare results, but when so many of the quality indicators point in the same direction, we can draw some meaningful conclusions. And the evidence here points to two conclusions we can accept with certainty: Canadians live longer (and by many criteria are healthier) than Americans, and Canadians are much happier with their health care system than Americans are with ours.

Death rates from heart disease are higher in the United States than in Canada. (In 1985, the United States suffered 434 deaths from heart disease per 100,000 population, significantly more than the 348 deaths per 100,000 in Canada.)[2]

Infant mortality rates are much lower in Canada. In 1988, Canada had an infant mortality rate of 7 deaths per 1,000 births. The United States infant mortality rate that year was 10 deaths per 1,000 births. In fact, infant mortality for *whites* in the United States is worse than for *all races* in Canada![3]

The United States ranks fifteenth in the proportion of babies born at low birthweight, a crucial risk factor for infant death and for mental and physical disability.[4]

Many factors are at work besides the health care system — poverty, drug addiction, education, and others — but no one can doubt that the high U.S. infant morbidity and infant mortality rates would be lower if prenatal care were better and more widely available.

Even the most basic health care is not reaching many of our kids. The incidence of major childhood diseases has increased in the United States since 1980, while the immunization rate has fallen. One out of five American two-year-olds is not fully protected against polio, rubella, mumps, or measles. The immunization rates in the United States for diphtheria, pertussis, and tetanus are half those of Western Europe or Canada.[5]

Canada has slightly fewer physicians per population than the United States. In 1990, Canada had a ratio of 448 people per physician, whereas the United States had 434 per physician.[6] But this does not lead to better access or better health in the United States than in Canada. For one thing, there are no out-of-pocket charges for Canadian patients, so there is not the economic incentive Americans commonly feel to delay visits to the doctor until they get sicker.

Even though Americans pay more for medical treatment, it can sometimes be lower quality than what Canadians get. Consider how highly specialized care is distributed. Canadians in need of specialized care are referred to medical centers of excellence, where specialist skills and technology are concentrated. Canadian patients are not charged for the state-of-the-art care they receive. Even their travel expenses are paid when these medical centers are not nearby.

In the United States, new technology is distributed to far more institutions, diluting the expertise required to get optimal results from complex equipment and procedures. A report in the *Annals of Internal Medicine* shows that more mammography machines are distributed in the United States than can be used efficiently.[7] This makes mammograms needlessly expensive. Even those women who have adequate insurance are hurt by the too-widespread diffusion of this technology, because quality control suffers. A report by the General Accounting Office, for example, recently found that mammography screening facilities that did a high volume of work were more likely to conform to quality standards than were those doing fewer mammograms.[8] For one thing, the number of mammogram machines sold has far outpaced the supply of certified radiological technologists available to help operate them. Dr. Robert McLelland of the University of North Carolina School of Medicine writes: "Less than 20 percent of the estimated total number of mammography units in the United States have been accredited!"[9]

One danger cited in the *Annals of Internal Medicine* report is an excessive number of false-positive results of mammogram readings.[10] That means unnecessary biopsy surgery for many women, with all the anxiety, discomfort, and risks associated with surgery.

Mammography is only one area where the costly over-distribution of high-tech medical systems has diminished the quality of care available to the American public. Another is heart bypass surgery.

The medical profession acknowledges that a hospital must perform a given number of bypass operations or other open-heart procedures each year to maintain a high standard of care. The American College of Surgeons has produced the following guidelines for open-heart surgery: "It is recognized that there is a critical density of case material that is required to maintain an adequate standard of practice. The performance of at least 150 open-heart operations per year by an independent team is desirable to maintain an adequate standard. A team may operate in more than one hospital. However, effective use of equipment and support personnel generally requires at least 150 cases per year in each hospital."[11]

Other medical authorities agree. There is general acceptance of the fact that hospitals that do more open-heart surgery have better outcomes, and there is a minimum volume of surgery a hospital must perform to maintain quality standards. The *New England Journal of Medicine* reported as early as 1979 that "the mortality of open-heart surgery, vascular surgery, transurethral resection of the prostate, and coronary bypass decreased with increasing number of operations. Hospitals in which 200 or more of these operations were done annually had death rates, adjusted for case mix, 25 to 41 percent lower than hospitals with lower volumes."[12]

The problem is this: as high-tech medical systems proliferate to more and more hospitals in the United States, allowing more hospitals to do open-heart surgery, the volume of surgery performed at some individual hospitals has dropped. The heart surgery business is being divided up among more hospitals, and quality of care has dropped as a result.

A well-documented example of this alarming trend comes from Phoenix, Arizona. Until 1985, the Arizona legislature prevented the haphazard proliferation of heart surgery technology to Arizona hospitals. Until 1985, hospitals had to demonstrate need for increased capacity before they could expand the expensive medical systems that support heart surgery.

But in March 1985, the legislature deregulated Arizona's

hospital industry. And Arizona's hospitals raced to get in on the profitable business of heart bypass surgery. Before the rules were lifted, seven hospitals in Phoenix and Tucson performed heart surgery; afterward, seventeen hospitals were in the market.

The losers were the patients. A special report by the *Phoenix Gazette* revealed that death rates for Medicare patients undergoing bypass surgery in Arizona jumped 35 percent between 1984 and 1986. The hospitals with the highest death rates were also the ones doing the lowest volumes of surgery. Reporter Brad Patten writes:

> Deregulation has spawned a group of seven hospitals with death rates exceeding ten percent for Medicare patients undergoing coronary artery bypass surgery, one of the most common major surgical procedures.
>
> Since deregulation, Medicare bypass patients in these low-volume hospitals have died at twice the rate of those in the state's busiest heart-surgery units. The odds of dying at higher-volume surgery units are unchanged.[13]

High-volume hospitals had 60 deaths per 1,000 procedures, while low-volume hospitals had 117 deaths per 1,000. Commenting on this result, Jonathan Showstack, associate professor of health policy at the University of California, San Francisco, said: "If you take 200 bypass patients from one hospital and divide them among two hospitals . . . all of those patients have a higher likelihood of dying or having a poor outcome."[14]

The motive behind the flood of new heart surgery centers is not the search for quality medical care, but the search for profits. New open-heart surgery centers quickly recoup their initial investments and go on to earn hefty profits. An open-heart surgery program in Arizona can generate profits of as much as $1.7 million a year, according to the *Gazette*.[15]

An ironic twist is that the overproliferation of high-tech medical procedures doesn't save money for the patients. Increased competition means the unnecessary duplication of very expensive equipment. The cost of that equipment is passed on to the consumer. The *Gazette* report pointed out that in January 1985, before Arizona's deregulation, the average cost of a bypass procedure in the state was $16,064. Two years later, after ten hospitals entered the bypass surgery market, the cost had jumped to $23,988.[16] Once again, consumers were paying more for their health care and getting less in terms of quality.

Sophisticated medical technology in Canada is concentrated in centers of excellence. Not every hospital is expected to provide every state-of-the-art procedure. The result is that those hospitals doing, say, organ transplants or heart valve surgery do a great deal of it—just like centers of excellence in the United States. This enables those centers to develop extensive experience and greater expertise. It means that virtually every Canadian has access to the best of the brightest doctors. (Coincidentally, it is also more efficient, and therefore less expensive, to organize care in this rational way.)

Medical outcomes are improved by this approach to organizing medicine sensibly. For example, Ontario has found that the concentration of neonatal intensive care in a few centers of excellence has led to the increased proficiency of the staffs of those units, because they have such extensive practical experience. In a National Public Radio interview on "All Things Considered," Dr. Martin Barkin, then Ontario's deputy health minister, said: "The survival of babies that come in at a pound or a pound and a half, some less than a pound, is entirely dependent on extremely sophisticated technology and very highly trained human resources: nurses, respiratory technologists, and so forth. You cannot have a functioning critical-care capacity for that in every hospital and maintain a level of skill and quality" (August 16, 1989).

Another measure of the dichotomy between cost and outcome is the solid support of Canadians for their national health insurance program and the overwhelming dissatisfaction among Americans with our balkanized private insurance system—despite the higher per capita spending on our side of the border.

A 1988 Harris poll found that only 10 percent of Americans think their system works "pretty well," while 89 percent think that the American health care system requires fundamental change or complete rebuilding. Meanwhile, 56 percent of Canadians think their system works "pretty well," and only 42 percent think it needs extensive reworking. The same poll showed that 61 percent of Americans would trade the U.S. health care system for the Canadian system, while only 37 percent would keep the status quo. Among Canadians, however, 95 percent said they would keep their own system, given the choice to trade with America; only 3 percent of Canadians preferred the American model.[17]

Poll data are one barometer for reading the support of Canadians for their health care system. Another is the depth of passion with which Canadians defend their health insurance program in the political arena. This was obvious during the 1989 parliamentary debate over Canada's free trade agreement with the United States. Opponents of the treaty nearly succeeded in killing it by arguing that the pact would destroy the Canadian health care system. Defeat of the agreement was only headed off at the last minute — and then only when the founders of the health care system themselves called on Canadians to recognize that the free trade agreement would not harm it.

All major Canadian political parties, representing the spectrum from left to right, support Canada's health insurance program wholeheartedly. Not to do so would be political suicide, because the approval of the Canadian public for their national health insurance runs very deep. Canadians love their health care system — because it works, and because they feel that they can afford it!

No matter how health care spending is compared, the United States spends more than Canada. Indeed, the United States spends more than anyone else.

As a proportion of gross national product (GNP), the United States spends more than Canada, more than England, more than Sweden, or Germany, or Japan. In 1989, the United States spent 11.6 percent of its GNP on health care, Canada only 8.9 percent.[18]

Per capita, the United States also spends more. In 1990, Americans spent an estimated $2,425 on health care for every man, woman, and child in the United States. In the same year, Canada spent only $1,888 (in U.S. dollars) for each Canadian. And for that price, every Canadian received excellent-quality care, whereas the United States, which spent 39 percent more, protected only a decreasing portion of our citizens. The Census Bureau found that more than sixty-three million Americans, mostly working people and their children, went without any health insurance at all for a month or more over a recent twenty-eight-month period. Tens of millions more are dangerously underinsured.[19]

The spending differential has increased steadily. That $2,425 per person the United States spent in 1990 was up from $1,016 just ten years earlier. The figure is expected to more than double again in another ten years, to $5,515 per person per year by the year 2000.

Robert Evans estimates that if the United States had been able to hold down growth in health spending to the level of growth Canada experienced between 1971 and 1987, we would have saved $450 per year per American, for a total annual savings of $100 billion.[20]

Americans are spending more for several reasons, and comparisons with the Canadian system are instructive. We pay exorbitant fees to specialists, and we have proportionately more specialists and fewer primary care physicians than the Canadians. We pay for extra layers of administrative red tape caused by the balkanized private insurance system, with 1,500 insurers instead of Canada's one per province. And the same overdistribution of technology that threatens quality also vastly increases costs.

Lesson 2: We Can *All* Have Quality *and* Affordability

It is possible to simultaneously ensure quality, control costs, and make health care available to everybody. Indeed, it may not in the long run be possible to achieve any one of these three goals without achieving all three: quality, availability, and cost control.

Canada is achieving all three, right now.

The ultimate guarantor of quality in the Canadian health system is its politicization. Unlike insurance company executives, legislators are directly responsible to the whole people. The government has to answer for every gap in quality control, every delay, every weakness in the system. And because the Canadian health system is universal, the entire electorate shares an interest in getting things fixed. Every Canadian feels that he or she has a stake in the system, a lot riding on its success.

Canadian construction workers never have to worry about whether they can afford to pay health insurance premiums, as do many of their American counterparts. Older Canadians do not live with perpetual fear that if they get sick, they might lose their home and savings. Canadian children reap the benefits of a system that guarantees the best care available, beginning with prenatal care.

Canadian medicine operates as social insurance, which is also the principle behind Social Security and Medicare in the United States. Canadian medical care is not "socialized medicine." Canadian doctors don't work for the government. Canadian doctors operate privately, just like American doctors. The only thing centralized is the administration of health insurance. And that centralization saves piles of money — enough to finance the high quality of health care that all Canadians receive without any copayments or deductibles. The centralized administration of health insurance also gives the provincial governments the tools to hold down hospital costs and medical fees.

Quality, accessibility, and cost control are intertwined concepts, each underpinning the other. They can't be separated. Together, they make possible the success of the Canadian health care system.

Canadians readily admit that they can only afford timely, high-quality universal care because they give sensible attention to cost containment.

Because all Canadians have access to care that is free at point of use, Canadians are more likely to receive health care on a timely basis than are the increasing number of middle-income Americans who feel the pressure of rapidly rising medical charges. In the United States, where diagnostic work and preventive care are expensive, many people have a powerful incentive to postpone or try to do without. With diseases such as diabetes, high blood pressure, and cancer, these delays can be deadly. At best, they can be expensive.

Getting sick people to the doctor in a timely fashion saves money and lives. But 40 percent of doctors responding to a recent poll of internists in the United States cited increasing numbers of patients delaying treatment or disregarding doctors' instructions for reasons of cost.

The motor of the Canadian system is patient need — *medical need* — instead of the need to earn profits, which is the catalyst for action in a system where many key decisions are made by hospital administrators and insurance companies.

And it is the commitment to universality and quality that underlie the ability of the system to rely on widespread and deep support for its decision-making processes and its funding.

As the United States confronts a crisis of health care cost, quality, and access, it is clear that — like the Canadians — solving any one requires solving the other two. Consider, for example, the crisis many cities face in emergency medicine. Trauma centers, unable to withstand the financial drain of increasing amounts of unreimbursed services (as increasing numbers of Americans are priced, or redlined, out of health insurance coverage), are shutting down. Providing unreimbursed emergency services is some drain on hospitals, but that is only the tip of the problem. For the seriously ill or injured, the emergency room is a gateway to lengthy stays in the hospital, also unreimbursed. And, denied access to primary care elsewhere, patients without health insurance frequently use the emergency room as their entry point, often after harmful delays that exacerbate their condition. One result is that the financial drain of operating an emergency room is increasing, convincing hospitals to shut them down. In cities all across the country, this endangers the lives of all citizens, regardless of their insurance coverage, as access to emergency rooms is cut by the cost of care for the uninsured. The only way we're ever going to make sure that there are adequate numbers of emergency rooms is to face up to the need to get the mushrooming crisis of the uninsured under control.

The realization we must achieve is that, in a complex technological society, holistic approaches to our problems are often the only workable approaches. Canada demonstrates that cost, quality, and access can only be addressed as a whole.

Lesson 3: We Can Get More Freedom of Choice Than We Have Now

Systems of universal access, such as Canada's national health insurance, can give patients and doctors far more freedom of choice than the system of health care financing now in place in the United States.

Canadians make their medical decisions free from worry about whether they can afford to pay for treatment. But they also have freedom to shop around and find a doctor they're comfortable with. They can get a second opinion — or a third — whenever they feel the need to, without worrying about extra expense. Patients in Canada decide on their medical treatment in consultation with the doctor of their choice. There is no third party in that decision-making process, no insurance company to approve or disapprove the decision, and no economic disincentive to seeking preventive care or timely diagnosis and treatment.

Canadian patients have complete freedom to choose their doctors. The patient decides what general practitioners or internists to consult, and how often.

And the freedom assured by Canadian health insurance extends beyond the health care marketplace into other areas of life. Canadians do not have to worry about losing their health protection if they want to (or are forced to) change jobs. They are guaranteed continuity of coverage; they never have to worry about preexisting conditions or waiting periods for new insurance coverage to kick in when they take a new job.

In contrast, the rising cost of health care in the United States, coupled with our haphazard system of financing that care, seriously limits the health care freedom of choice of Americans. Before Americans go to the doctor, they must do mental calculations to work out whether their insurance covers the visit. (If they have no private insurance, there is a chance they will have recourse to Medicaid, if they are poor enough to meet strict eligibility limits.) In practice, many Americans will just not feel free to seek medically necessary care — especially preventive care.

If you have private insurance, you have to check to see whether your insurance is accepted by the doctor of your choice, and whether the insurance covers the procedure your doctor suggests. You must then work out whether you can afford the deductible and the copayments. All of this, in practice, limits your freedom of choice in the health care marketplace. And, unlike the limits that cost places on your freedom of choice in

the purchase of other services or goods, you are not choosing
between varying degrees of luxury. You are choosing, quite simply, whether to get the care you need in a timely manner.

The greater freedom of the Canadian patient is achieved
without restricting the freedom of the Canadian doctor. Physicians in Canada are not restricted in their daily practice. Their
relationship with the provincial government is strictly financial:
the province is the insurer, not the micro-manager of health care.
And Canadian doctors don't have to answer to insurance company gatekeepers for every decision they make, as American
doctors have to.

The insurance company clearance system in the United
States is not at all related to quality control. Quite the contrary.
The private insurance company gatekeepers are not seeking to
ensure that all medically necessary treatment is performed; they
are in place only to limit the financial liability of the insurance
companies.

Lesson 4: We Can Cut Red Tape

It is possible to reduce the costly and annoying paperwork that
plagues the private United States insurance system. Doctors,
as well as patients, will appreciate the result.

In the United States, there are 1,500 private and public
health insurers, each with its own rules, regulations, and administrative processes. In Canada, most health care bills are
paid by one of eleven entities: the ten provincial governments
and, in the territories, the federal government. Canadians go
to private doctors, just as we do, but there is only one insurance plan in each province. Everybody belongs to it.

One result is that the paperwork and red tape that burden the United States health care system are dramatically less
in Canada.

The United States spends massively more on administering health care, per capita, than Canada does. Robert Evans
writes that in 1985, the United States spent $95 for every man,
woman, and child in America on insurance company overhead
alone. This money did not go to buy health care; instead, it

went to paper shuffling and other administrative waste. Meanwhile, the Canadians spent only $18 per person.[21]

We can also compare overhead spending as a percentage of our countries' total health spending. In 1987, Canada spent just 1 percent of its health dollar on administration. Americans, whose health spending was much greater to start with, expended at least 7 percent spending on administration, and some experts put that figure at 10 percent or higher! And the more the insurance companies try to boost profits by limiting their liabilities through cost shifting, the more we wind up spending on health care administration overall, because cost shifting inevitably adds to paperwork.

U.S. experience shows that consolidating the financing of health care can save huge sums of money by cutting overhead. Only 2.7 percent of Medicare and Medicaid spending goes for administrative costs. Compare that with private small-market insurance plans, where an average of one-third of premiums go to pay for bloated overhead, including advertising, agent commissions, and profits.

The current crazy-quilt health insurance system spawns diverse and duplicative payment rules, differing rates, myriad separate utilization review systems, complex and costly eligibility determinations, and high marketing costs. Americans, in effect, pay what one economist has described as a "plurality tax" on all health services.

Administrative waste helps make health care unaffordable for millions. And it directs resources into paperwork that would better be spent on raising quality.

The Canadian solution is not the only way to get administrative red tape under control. But one key lesson is that red tape should and can be cut and that it can be done through at least some degree of consolidation of the health care financing system.

If insurance company red tape and nearly endless paperwork drives patients crazy, pity the physicians who have to deal with this red tape throughout their workday.

That is one reason that the American College of Physicians, the second largest physicians' association in the United

States, with 68,000 members, came out in favor of comprehensive health reform.

The fact is that most Canadian doctors are happy with their system. They don't have the hassle of filling out reams of paperwork for a thousand different insurance companies. They don't have to worry about getting paid. They don't have to screen patients for the ability to pay. They don't have to see their patients denied necessary care because of anomalies in the insurance system.

A measure of Canadian doctors' feelings about their health care system is the number of physicians who leave Canada to practice elsewhere. Fewer than 1 percent of physicians have left Canada annually since national health insurance was enacted. This is a very low number for any Canadian profession. Canadian professions are susceptible to what has been called the "Gretzky effect," where the best in any field are enticed across the border to the United States by the lure of big money, fame, and fortune, as Canadian hockey star Wayne Gretzky was attracted to Los Angeles. A figure of less than 1 percent emigration may be explained by nonprofessional motives alone, such as emigration after a cross-border marriage, climatic preferences, or old-fashioned wanderlust.

The number of physicians entering Canada annually has exceeded the number leaving in every year since 1986. So many doctors have tried to enter Canada, in fact, that the government limited the number of visas made available to them.

Another measure of the success of the Canadian health care system in making the practice of medicine attractive is that Canadian college students are clamoring to get into medical school. For each position open in Canadian medical schools, there were more than four applicants. That compares with 1.7 applicants per position in the United States.[22]

All these data point to one conclusion: Canadian doctors like their health care system. It gives them freedoms that American physicians don't have. It frees them to make medical decisions with their patients without interference from a thousand insurance companies. And it frees them from the administrative hassle that eats up so much of an American doctor's day.

In short, it frees them to do what their education prepared them to do: practice medicine.

Lesson 5: States May Have a Leadership Role to Play in Health Care Financing Reform

Just as Canada's health reform began in Saskatchewan, there may be a role for states to experiment with financing mechanisms, finding what works and what doesn't.

Canada, like the United States, operates under a federal system. Canada's provinces vary greatly in terms of population density and other demographic characteristics, as do our states. And they vary politically at least as much as our states do.

In Canada, public health insurance got an early start. In the prairie provinces, with sparse populations of family farmers, the need for public intervention in health care delivery was felt early on. In order to get doctors to come to rural areas to serve the farm population, villages got together to hire municipal doctors. In the prairies, towns have contracted to provide this form of health care delivery for local residents since before World War I.

The prairie provinces also created early prototypes of involvement in hospital policy. Alberta and Saskatchewan passed laws in the 1910s enabling rural towns to establish municipal hospitals.

But it didn't stop there in Saskatchewan. The accession to power of a prairie populist party — similar to populist parties in Minnesota and the Dakotas — set the stage for major changes in health care financing in the postwar decades of the 1950s to the 1970s. The populists' initial interest in health care was spurred by the mood of a public fed up with hardships inflicted by years of depression and war, and by the instincts of the party's Hubert Humphrey–like leader, T. C. Douglas.

A province or a state can be a huge laboratory for testing ideas. That was the role Saskatchewan played. When the province inaugurated its provincial hospital insurance plan, health policy people from all over Canada flocked there to observe the strengths and weaknesses of the new program. The same thing happened again, later, when the province enacted a public medical insurance program.

Perhaps more important, politicians elsewhere in Canada watched — and learned — as the populists in Saskatchewan successfully maneuvered through the political minefields.

The fact is that Saskatchewan had more creative political leadership than the Canadian federal government did at that time. But the politicians in Ottawa learned from the prairie populists, and what started as a radical experiment in one province soon became the political mainstream nationally.

Lesson 6: Single Tier Works Best

A single-tier social insurance system creates a political constituency for high-quality health care that cannot be achieved in multitier systems.

The most popular federal programs in the United States are Medicare and Social Security. They hold a special place in the American political realm, as shown by the outcry when Social Security got into trouble in the late 1970s and early 1980s and when the White House tried to reduce Medicare benefits in 1990.

One reason Medicare and Social Security are so popular is that they're so fair. You receive benefits after you've earned the privilege through years of honest work. Everyone who works pays in. Everyone who pays in earns the right to take out.

Take Social Security as an example. Because every American is eligible to receive the benefits of Social Security, the program has a very broad base of support. Its support is not confined to the poor or the wealthy, or to the residents of any particular area or the workers in any particular industry. Social Security is an insurance program for all Americans, and all kinds of Americans support it passionately. Almost every family has somebody now paying in; almost every family has somebody now drawing benefits.

The great popularity of Social Security and the breadth of its support base mean that politicians are under tremendous pressure to protect it and improve it. Politicians heed their constituents, and voters in every congressional district in America support Social Security. Politicians are blasted with complaints whenever there is a hint that Social Security might be endangered or trimmed. And the complaints come from the whole spectrum of a politician's constituency: the well-to-do, the poor, and (most important, politically) the middle-income. Broad-based programs like Social Security thrive because their breadth of support gives them a built-in incentive for politicians to protect and improve them.

Most politicians know they have to be seen as protectors of Social Security. Even ideological right-wingers don't usually try a direct attack. They may believe in their hearts that all government programs are bad and that Social Security is as bad as the rest of them. But the political tactic they use is to split the program's broad base of support by trying to cut rich seniors out of the program, or allow the rich to opt out.

If the opponents of Social Security could succeed in doing this, the program would be seriously threatened. By removing the economically better-off from the program, they would weaken political support for the program among its most politicized constituency. There would be less political pressure on politicians to maintain and improve the program. The end result would be a lower-quality program, as money is diverted from it to other interests of the highly politicized groups that have been excluded from it. You end up with a two-tier system, where some Americans are excluded from the program altogether, and those who are left get less protection because they have less political clout. One important lesson we can learn from Canada is that this same principle of political-strength-through-unity can be applied to the health care system. Canadians like and support their health care system because they have a vested interest in it. They like it because it's fair. And that very fairness, rooted in universality, ensures a uniform, high-quality standard of care for all Canadians. As far as health care goes, all Canadians are in the same boat, and for that reason, the boat is kept in well-maintained, seaworthy condition.

The lesson for American health reformers is this: even if your goal in reforming health care is to improve the lot of the poor and the unfortunate, the best way to do that is to achieve — as nearly as possible in our political context — a one-

tier system of health care. Reform must serve the interests of
the middle class if it is to have a politically secure future.

To see the truth of this, we need only look as far as our
current Medicaid program. Medicaid was designed to be a medical safety net for the poorest and most vulnerable Americans.
But Medicaid patients still face enormous obstacles to getting
the care they need. Benefits vary wildly from state to state. Many
desperately needy persons receive no help at all. Others are entitled to help—theoretically—but cannot find a doctor who accepts patients on Medicaid's skimpy fee schedule. Many thousands who should be eligible for Medicaid help do not receive
it because of the cumbersome process of applying for it, or because it is perceived as "charity." All these Americans and their
families would be better served under a one-tier system offering excellent medical care to everyone—rich and poor alike.

From a realistic political standpoint, however, we may
not in the near future be able to achieve the sort of single-tier
system that the Canadians have. But the larger the pool of
Americans covered, even in a multitiered system, the closer we
come to achieving the political strength of a one-tier system.
If, for instance, employer-based financing reform covers all
workers and their families and provides a unified publicly sponsored, privately operated program for all the self-employed and
the unemployed, including the current beneficiaries of Medicaid,
then we would have created a program broad enough to protect
quality politically. We would also have achieved real cost cutting through administrative savings and tough bargaining with
providers.

Lesson 7: Artificial Coverage Limits Don't Work

Over the years the Canadians have been shaping their health
care system, the very clear trend has been toward elimination
of artificial limits on health care protection. They have found
that protecting people over sixty-five, but not under, or covering acute care, but not chronic care, or making nursing homes
available, but not homemaker services, does not serve a useful
social purpose and is not economically justified.

Three of the basic tenets of Canadian health care — comprehensiveness, universality, and portability — address this question of where the limits should be.

Canada draws those limits wide.

The Canada Health Act of 1984 enshrines in law the principle that health care be comprehensive. That is, all medically necessary care must be provided under the provincial health insurance plans. The effect of this provision is to prevent arbitrary discrimination of the sort that appears in private health insurance in the United States all the time. For example, in the United States, private insurers often place an arbitrary limit on coverage of mental health care, or on the amount of help available to patients with certain disorders, such as Alzheimer's disease, that require a great deal of nursing, homemaker, or custodial service. By and large, these distinctions would not be made in Canada.

Are there de facto limits in the Canadian system that are not related to medical necessity? Are such limits inherent in any system that relies on global budgeting? Critics of the Canadian health care system insist that these limits do exist. Advocates of the Canadian system, including Robert Evans, Orvill Adams, and most other Canadian health economists, argue that there is a conscious and continuing effort to eliminate these limits — which, they contend, is one reason why Canada spends more than most other nations on health care. And the fact is that Canadian patients do not feel that their health care system functions badly or denies them easy access to necessary care.

The Canada Health Act requires that the provincial health insurance plans provide universal coverage. That means that everybody living in the province must be protected. There are no rules discriminating against anyone on the basis of occupation, health history, marital status, employment status, length of coverage, place of residence, or ability to pay.

The Canada Health Act also requires that there are no fees for service, of any sort, including balance billing — thus eliminating disincentives to utilization that impact most heavily on the most vulnerable. There is no income testing to keep anyone from participating in the system. And the Canada Health

Act also guarantees portability, so that Canadians are not excluded from coverage when they move from job to job, from
one end of the country to the other.

Canadians feel, quite rightly, that any artificial limits on
health care work against achieving the goal of a healthy society.

In the United States, the effect of artificial limits on health
coverage is to stop some people from getting health care they
need. Our health care financing system places medically un-
justified limits on the care you get. Doing this serves no useful
social purpose. It doesn't discourage people from getting sick
or needing care. Limiting health care doesn't work like a "sin
tax" on alcohol or cigarettes, because illness isn't a sin.

The only case for any of these limits would be cost. But
the Canadian model demonstrates the irony that *some* limits on
care wind up costing Americans money. We have seen how the
way we finance health care, with all of its arbitrary limits on
protection, costs vastly more than the Canadian system, where
everyone gets the care they need. And the scaling down of unnecessary limits is part of the reason that the Canadian system
is so much cheaper to administer and more amenable to cost-
effective preventive care.

Lesson 8: Comprehensive Long Term Care
Protection Strengthens Families

It is striking how comprehensive long term care protection that
includes extensive home- and community-based services strengthens Canadian families by making it possible for generations
to help each other.

The story of a man I will call "Mr. Smith" shows how
the different parts of the health insurance plan in most Canadian
provinces work together to help heal individuals and families.

Mr. Smith is an elderly widower from a small town in
remote northern British Columbia. He fell ill while visiting his
son's family in Victoria, the provincial capital, in September
1990. After medical treatment and a joint medical/social work
assessment by provincial long term care specialists, it became
clear that Mr. Smith's clinical condition was worsened by depres-

sion, poor nutrition, and alcohol abuse. And it was equally clear that these problems were the results of isolation and loneliness.

Under the circumstances, the best thing possible would be for Mr. Smith to move in with his children in Victoria rather than returning to his isolated home in the north. The old man's son and daughter-in-law wanted desperately to help, but they both work full time. In addition, they have one child in high school and two more in grade school. If Mr. Smith were to move in with them (which everyone wanted), the family would need help looking after Mr. Smith during the day, when no adult family member could be at home with him.

The province's long term care program provided three and a half hours of home support, five days a week, to help Mr. Smith get around and prepare his meals. In addition, the province installed a medical alert system in the family's home.

Mr. Smith's mental and physical status have greatly improved—largely because he could stay with his family and not have to choose between living alone or being institutionalized. The government's help made it possible for the family to do all it could, and the province's help came at a financial cost significantly lower than the cost of institutionalization.

The "Smith" family story is important to us because almost every American family ultimately faces a long term care crisis.

Nearly one of every two people over the age of sixty-five will eventually spend some time in a nursing home. One in five will spend a year or more in a nursing home. Nine million Americans who aren't in nursing homes required community-based long term care in 1989.[23]

Millions of Americans who may not need daily physician services *do* need day-to-day help with the everyday chores of life, such as cooking, cleaning, bathing, toileting, or getting around.

In the United States, the need for long term care can mean more than the loss of independence. In the United States, the need for long term care often brings financial disaster.

A 1988 Harris poll found that 82 percent of adults surveyed could not afford to pay for long term care.[24] A year in a nursing home now costs an average of more than $30,000. (It costs $50,000 or more in our larger cities.) In some states, Medicaid will pay for nursing home care—but only after the patient has spent herself or himself into poverty in order to qualify. And help with home care is not available to most Americans who need it to remain independent.

Private insurance companies have been trying to enter the long term care market. But because the risks of insuring the elderly are high, the policies available are very expensive. A 1990 study by Families USA Foundation showed that 84 percent of Americans aged sixty-five to seventy-nine cannot afford the average basic nursing home care insurance policy, and 73 percent cannot afford even the lowest-priced policy.[25] In point of fact, private insurance pays for less than 2 percent of long term care costs.

In addition, the marketing of private long term care insurance is rank with abuse. Many of the policies that have been sold are so riddled with loopholes and exclusions as to make them virtually worthless.

But the real and tragic impact of the long term care crisis in the United States is on the families of those needing care. Long term care can drive a family into bankruptcy. Right now, of the $65 billion in total nursing home costs in the United States, nearly half is being paid, often at great sacrifice, by American families. And home care is a burden borne almost entirely, at great sacrifice, by families.[26]

The vast majority of long term care is provided by family and friends. Many of these people are themselves elderly or in poor health. Often, the chief caregiver is the eldest daughter or daughter-in-law.

Being a caregiver is no small task. Four out of five are responsible for caregiving seven days a week. The ongoing mental and physical demands of looking after a long term care patient are enough to put the strongest, most loving persons under intolerable stress.

When the stresses of providing care are added to the financial impossibility of meeting the cost of care, the burden can become unbearable. Most women today work at paid jobs outside the home, but women are still expected to provide long term care for family members who may need it, while bringing home an income at the same time. This can be more than even today's "superwomen" can manage.

Of long term caregivers with jobs outside the home, about 20 percent have had to cut down their paid work hours. Another 20 percent have had to take unpaid leave. Some 25 percent have had to rearrange their work schedules. And 10 percent have had to quit their jobs.[27]

Even giving these caregivers a little time off would help immensely. "Respite care," or temporary care provided by outsiders to allow the usual caregivers a brief rest, provides much-needed breathing space. But many caregivers cannot afford respite care, often at a cost of upward of $100 a day.

Family members who care for chronically ill loved ones do so out of love, and because they believe it's their responsibility. Family caregivers tend to be strong people. But even they can be stretched to the breaking point by the financial hardship on top of the other emotional burdens that go with caregiving.

For example, we can look at the "Wagner" family, who care for Jim Wagner's mother in their home. The elder Mrs. Wagner suffers from advanced Alzheimer's disease. She needs twenty-four-hour supervision. The family has not had even a week's vacation in several years. Why? The cost of caring for Jim's mother eats up most of their disposable income. It would be possible for the family to scrape together enough for a week at a nearby seashore, if they could take Jim's mother along. But they are afraid to take her away with them, because travel disorients her. The one time they tried to take her to the beach, they found that they could not leave her unsupervised for even a moment. When they so much as turned their back, she started eating sand and pebbles. Now they feel they cannot travel with her, because they are afraid they will not be able to supervise her adequately. But they cannot leave her home, either, because of the expense of respite care.

Respite care in their area costs $100 a day or more. A week's trip would cost them $700 for care for Jim's mother, before they ever set foot out the door. With all the other expenses of caring for her, that is a price they will never be able to afford.

(In places where affordable respite care is available, such as most of Canada, its value to families is twofold. It provides much-needed opportunities for the caregiver to carry on a normal life. But it also relieves the stress most caregivers feel that they are "out there all alone," that there is no backup if an emergency strikes. Just knowing that respite care is available is at least as much help as the respite care itself.)

Many families who have to meet educational costs for their children while providing long term care for their parents find themselves in desperate straits. And — as America ages — their numbers are growing daily.

The long term care problem has Americans worried. Before the 1988 presidential election, a survey by Peter D. Hart Research Associates asked voters aged eighteen to forty-four to name the most important domestic issues for the next president to address. Long term care was the no. 1 issue, eliciting more concern than the drug epidemic, environmental problems, education, or crime. A similar survey by Hamilton, Frederick & Schneiders asked voters above the age of forty-five to rank their priorities for government spending. Again, long term care was the no. 1 priority, outranking the environment, farm programs, aid to the homeless, and defense.[28]

In 1992, a Gallup Poll done for the American Medical Association found that only 13 percent of Americans were very confident they would be able to pay for long term care.[29] And a 1991 survey of New Hampshire voters by Lauer, Lalley & Associates found 60 percent of those living in *high-income households* worried about affording a long term care crisis.[30] All of that underlies the 1987 finding by RL Associates of Princeton, New Jersey, that the vast majority of adult Americans (a proportion ranging from 81 percent of those aged forty to forty-nine to 92 percent of those aged eighteen to twenty-nine) favored government action on long term care.[31]

American popular support for government intervention in the long term care crisis is overwhelming. It is difficult to find another issue where there is so much agreement. Even if it means a new tax dedicated to this purpose, Americans want long term care protection.

Of American voters surveyed, 76 percent were willing to pay higher taxes to fund a federal long term care protection program. On this question, every group surveyed agreed. No matter what the respondents' income or age, a majority in every category said they would be willing to pay higher taxes if doing so would relieve them of the burden of paying for long term care. The poll confirmed that long term care is as important to younger voters as to older Americans, because long term care is a problem that impacts powerfully on entire families.

In Canada, public protection for long term care needs is strengthening families by giving them the tools they need to look after one another.

In most Canadian provinces, long term care is an important part of the health insurance program. Seven of Canada's ten provinces, representing 95 percent of Canada's entire population, provide nursing home insurance to all adults. And nonmedical home care is provided in all provinces. Canada invests in home care for her chronically ill, including help with chores such as housework and laundry as well as home visits by medical practitioners.

Canadian long term care specialists continue to develop innovative ways of meeting chronic care needs and keeping long term care patients functioning in the community.

In Victoria, British Columbia, for example, there is a long term care Quick Response Team (QRT) operating sixteen hours a day, 365 days a year. This project was started to prevent unnecessary hospitalizations of frail elderly residents of the capital region. Often, when an older person falls or has some other accident or illness and must visit an emergency room for urgent care, there is a dilemma. The person has no medical need to be admitted to the hospital, but the person can't go home alone if there is nobody there who can help for a few days. In the past, this situation often led to older persons being hospitalized unnecessarily, disrupting their lives, and slowing their recovery.

But now, in Victoria, doctors and emergency room staff can get help for these people. Seven days a week, until late at night, doctors or emergency room personnel can call the QRT

and get immediate emergency home support help so that patients can go home instead of having to be admitted to the
hospital.

The QRT has recently been expanded, so that it can also
be called on to provide temporary support when an elderly person is released from the hospital. In the gap of a few days after
discharge from the hospital, but before standard home care programs can be arranged, the QRT steps into the breach.

The QRT provides physiotherapy, homemaking assistance, and even equipment such as walkers and railings for the
bathroom.

This is the sort of humane, practical thinking that helps
the Canadians get more out of their health care dollars. It relieves
individuals, families — and hospital budgets — all at the same
time.

But the most striking aspect of the long term care system
in Canada — and its most important lesson for us — is the way
in which it reinforces family values and strengthens family bonds,
by making it financially possible for families to help themselves.

Lesson 9: Health Care Reform
Can Spark a Sense of Pride

When the health care system consistently provides access to high-
quality care, it can be a source of civic pride to a society. People in the United States don't need to be told that their health
care system is not what it should be. They know that. They know
they are paying more and more for the health care they get.
And they know that other countries are getting more for their
money than we are. That's why 61 percent of Americans would
trade the U.S. health care system for the Canadian one right
now.

Just like most Americans, Canadians think their country
is the best place to live for a bunch of reasons. Unlike Americans, however, Canadians cite health care as a prime reason.
Robert Evans has pointed out that Canadians get a certain satisfaction from knowing that, as far as health care goes, they "have
got it right." He likens the Canadians' pride in their health care

system (as compared with the U.S. system) to the satisfaction they would get from beating the Russians at hockey.

Evans also shows how the Canadian health care system belongs to the Canadians. It was shaped through the open, responsive Canadian democratic process. It reflects Canada's highest ideals: egalitarianism, cooperation, peace, order, and security.

If the health care system of a society is a mirror reflecting that society's ideals, what home truths do we learn from a look at the health care mess in the United States? It is no surprise we turn away, our civic pride shaken.

What American politician could run for office — as Canadian politicians do — by pointing with pride at the success of the health care system?

There are those who argue, Robert Evans most prominent among them, that the health care financing systems of Canada and the United States reflect the political realities of our two societies, the greater trust that Canadians place in government. But it may well be that — as Ian McKinnon argues — the political realities are in part shaped by our respective health care financing systems: that the success of Canada's health system inspires respect for government in a society that otherwise shares the healthy North American skepticism toward government.

The success of Canadian health care is itself one of the strongest arguments for the efficacy of government intervention to solve the real-life problems of ordinary Canadians. In fact, given the greater centrifugal forces of Canadian nationhood, in a divided land that did not even have a national flag until recently and still is in the process of establishing a permanent federal constitution, the health care system serves as a powerful force for national unity and national pride.

The lesson for us is that the American political system — as well as our health care system — may be strengthened by the progress we make together as a society in reforming the financing of health.

There is no reason why we, too, could not eventually look with pride on a health care system that — like the Canadian system — "gets it right."

Lesson 10: Doctors Can Earn a Decent Living
Without Billing Some Patients More Than Others

Balance billing is the practice whereby patients are billed above and beyond what the health insurance plan pays for a given service. It allows doctors to charge some patients more than others.

Balance billing is common in the United States. But in Canada, the practice was completely stopped by 1987, pursuant to the 1984 passage of the Canada Health Act. The act provided for federal funding to be cut from any provincial health programs where balance billing occurred.

But Canadian doctors make an excellent living — the best of any profession in the country.

In the United States, doctors make five to six times the average industrial wage. In Canada, doctors do only slightly less well: physicians' incomes are four to five times the average industrial wage. (Part of the difference is the result of the higher proportion of specialists in the United States and the higher proportion of primary care physicians north of the border.)

How can it be that, although Canadian doctors are no longer allowed to pad their incomes with balance billing, they still make very comfortable salaries that, for general practitioners and some specialists, are nearly on the scale of their American counterparts? There are several reasons.

For one thing, Canadian doctors don't have the expense of having to employ large billing staffs just to keep up with the paperwork.

Canadian doctors don't have to deal with the administrative nightmare of coping with 1,500 insurers, each with its own system of paperwork. Canadian doctors only have to bill one payer: the provincial health insurance system.

Canadian doctors are paid more quickly than American doctors. Canadian health care providers receive payment for their services in about 30 days. American health care providers wait between 60 and 120 days for payment, or even longer. American doctors have to go to great lengths to collect some bills, and some bills are never paid. Canadian doctors, on the other hand, are guaranteed payment for their services.

(Canadian doctors also enjoy the fact that the doctor-patient relationship isn't compromised by financial considerations. Canadian doctors never have to perform "wallet biopsies" on their patients to determine whether the patients can pay before treatment is even rendered.)

The Canadians thought — correctly — that balance billing erodes the quality of care available under a health insurance plan. It weakens the political consensus that forms in support of a one-tier system of care. And balance billing inhibits some people from getting care they need, by making that care more expensive.

Balance billing inflates the cost of administering a health insurance system. Instead of one payer with one billing procedure, you have as many payers as there are patients. This multiplies the paperwork and red tape enormously.

Balance billing also allows health care providers to escape attempts to limit health care inflation. When there is one payer, the health insurance plan, the plan can control costs by using its monopsony power to limit the fees it will pay. With balance billing, the insurance plan can try to hold down costs, but the care providers will simply exact the difference from patients who are balance billed.

Throughout Canada, in the early days of public health insurance, physicians used to be allowed to charge patients extra fees over and above those which would be reimbursed by the public insurance plan. But one by one, the provinces came to the conclusion that balance billing led to two problems. First, provincial administrators felt that balance billing made it impossible to control health costs. Second, balance billing seemed to split the Canadian public into two camps: the "haves," who could afford better-quality care, and the "have-nots," who, unable to pay extra, found themselves second-rate citizens who had to take whatever quality of care was offered to them. For many Canadians, balance billing threatened their access to the system at all, since a needed service might not even be offered except with a hefty additional fee, not covered by the provincial insurance.

This is why, beginning with Nova Scotia, all the provinces

outlawed the practice of balance billing. (The Canada Health
Act of 1984 tied federal funding to provincial elimination of
balance billing, completing the movement to a single-tier system.) The old practice had endangered the quality and availability of care for all Canadians, at the same time as it had made
cost containment impossible. Therefore, the Canadians aban-
doned it.

Underlying the decision to eliminate balance billing in
Canada is an ideological commitment to egalitarianism. As
Canada's former minister of National Health and Welfare, Perrin Beatty, put it: "It never struck me that anybody would feel
it was appropriate to buy better service or that someone could
jump the line as a result of having money. In Canada, we believe deeply that just as equal treatment under the law is essential, equality in terms of service for health care is a human entitlement."

Conversely, the ideological underpinning of the practice
of balance billing is the notion that ability to pay should determine one's right to live in health.

Lesson 11: National Health Reform
Doesn't Have to Be Done All at Once

We can build on what we have and improve as we go — as
Canada did. A national health care financing system doesn't suddenly appear in mature, final form, like Athena from the head
of Zeus. It evolves gradually, building on what is already in
place. The breadth of services grows. Reform may begin in one
geographical area, spreading to others as its success is confirmed.
Both of these evolutionary processes are healthy, perhaps even
necessary; both are, in fact, part of the Canadian experience.

Canada's national health insurance developed into its
present form over a span of decades, beginning in one province,
adding services incrementally, achieving its current status gradually. And, despite its successes, the evolution continues. Canadians expect that the system will continue to grow and improve,
and policy makers look forward to learning from experiments
(and American experiences) in managed care, community health

centers, and new techniques for managing the distribution of new technologies.

And at each step of this evolutionary process, Canada built on foundations already in place. The early hospital insurance plan developed in Saskatchewan in the 1940s built on experience with municipality-based hospital and doctor plans. The later nationwide plan drew much from the experience of Saskatchewan. Similarly, the nationwide medical insurance program of 1968 built on what had worked in the provinces' earlier attempts, which, in turn, had their roots in various health insurance models dating back to 1914.

Throughout this evolutionary process, Canada kept and developed the strong points of its health care system: an excellent medical infrastructure based on independent doctors and hospitals, and increasing reliance on a social insurance approach to funding.

The United States can glean this lesson from the Canadian experience: health care financing reform is an evolutionary process.

In fact, the United States has a long history of public involvement in health care financing, including Hill-Burton aid for hospital construction, distinguished medical research programs such as those of the National Institutes of Health, the Public Health Service, and, of course, Medicare and Medicaid. The U.S. government already offers federal public insurance for treatment of severe kidney disease. The government realizes that dialysis and related treatments are too expensive to be borne by most private individuals, but that the therapy is of such obvious value that it must be made available. The solution, as Congress has publicly decided, is social insurance.

We also have Medicare and Medicaid insurance for vulnerable populations — the elderly, the very poor, the disabled, and, most recently, moderate income children. These programs are analogous to the services provided under Saskatchewan's Health Services Act of 1945 — a law that proved to be a milestone on the road to public health insurance in the province.

Like Canada, the United States doesn't necessarily have to begin with action entirely at the federal level. Various states

are experimenting with health insurance programs with interesting features that might be suitable for adaptation to the needs
of the whole nation.

And, like Canada, the United States can adapt as we go,
keeping what works for us and changing what doesn't. The notion that we might adopt wholesale the system that Canada or
any other country uses is unrealistic. While we need comprehensive reform as rapidly as possible, reform in the United States
may come in stages — as it has in Canada.

That is why it may well be that the lessons we learn from
the Canadian experience may drive us down a different path
to achieving the results that the Canadians achieved on their
road to reform: a path as distinctly American as theirs has been
distinctly Canadian.

Notes

Chapter One

1. G. J. Schieber and J. P. Poullier, "Trends in International Health Care Spending," *Health Affairs,* 1987, *6*(3), 105; Organization for Economic Cooperation and Development (OECD), *Financing and Delivering Health Care,* OECD Social Policy Studies, no. 4 (Paris: OECD, 1987); A. J. Culyer, *Health Expenditures in Canada: Myth and Reality, Past and Future* (Toronto: Canadian Tax Foundation, 1988).
2. T. R. Marmor, "Doctors, Politics and Pay Disputes: Pressure Group Politics Revisited," in T. R. Marmor (ed.), *Political Analysis and American Medical Care: Essays* (Cambridge, England: Cambridge University Press, 1983); W. A. Glaser, *Paying the Doctor* (Baltimore, Md.: Johns Hopkins University Press, 1970).
3. T. R. Marmor, "Comparative Politics and Health Policies: Notes on Benefits, Costs, Limits," in Marmor, *Political Analysis and American Medical Care.*
4. M. G. Taylor, *Health Insurance and Canadian Public Policy* (Montreal: McGill-Queen's University Press, 1978); M. G. Taylor, "The Canadian Health Care System 1974–1984," in R. G. Evans and G. L. Stoddart (eds.), *Medicare at Matu-*

rity: Achievements, Lessons and Challenges (Calgary: University of Calgary Press for the Banff Centre, 1986); R. Fein, *Medical Care, Medical Costs: The Search for a Health Insurance Policy* (Cambridge, Mass.: Harvard University Press, 1986).

5. Schieber and Poullier, "Trends in International Health Care Spending"; OECD, *Financing and Delivering Health Care.*

6. S. Heiber and R. Deber, "Banning Extra-Billing in Canada: Just What the Doctor Didn't Order," *Canadian Public Policy,* 1987, *13*(1), p. 62.

7. Royal Commission on Health Services (Hall Commission), *Report,* vol. 1 (Ottawa: The Queen's Printer, 1964), esp. chapter. 1.

8. A. Enthoven, "Managed Competition in Health Care and the Unfinished Agenda," *Health Care Financing Review,* Annual Supplement, 1986, p. 105.

9. J. P. Poullier, personal communication subsequent to the OECD study of international health care financing and delivery systems.

10. Culyer, *Health Expenditures in Canada.*

11. M. L. Barer, R. G. Evans, and R. J. Labelle, "Fee Controls as Cost Control: Tales from the Frozen North," *The Milbank Quarterly,* 1988, *66*(1), pp. 1–64.

12. U. E. Reinhardt, "Resource Allocation in Health Care: The Allocation of Lifestyles to Providers." *Milbank Quarterly,* 1987,*65*(2), p. 153.

13. A. S. Detsky, S. R. Stacey, and C. Bombardier, "The Effectiveness of a Regulatory Strategy in Containing Hospital Costs: The Ontario Experience, 1967–1981," *New England Journal of Medicine,* 1983, *309*(3), pp. 151–159; M. L. Barer and R. G. Evans, "Riding North on a Southbound Horse? Expenditures, Prices, Utilization, and Incomes in the Canadian Health Care System," in R. G. Evans and G. L. Stoddart (eds.), *Medicare at Maturity: Achievements, Lessons and Challenges* (Calgary: University of Calgary Press for the Banff Centre, 1986).

14. D. Feeny, G. Guyatt, and P. Tugwell, *Health Care Technology: Effectiveness, Efficiency, and Public Policy* (Montreal: Institute for Research on Public Policy, 1986).

Chapter Two

1. L. Harris and Associates, "1987 Health Care Outlook Annual Report: Results and Implications of Two National Surveys," Sept. 1987.
2. American Medical Association, *Board of Trustees Report* (Chicago: American Medical Association, June 1989), p. 94.
3. Health and Welfare Canada, "Health Sector in Canada — Fact Sheets", unbound fact sheets produced by the Policy, Planning and Information Dissemination Unit, Ottawa, 1989, p. 2.
4. Health and Welfare Canada, *National Health Expenditures in Canada 1970–1982* (Ottawa: Policy, Planning and Information Dissemination Unit, 1984), pp. 1–9; Health and Welfare Canada, "Health Expenditures in Canada — Fact Sheets," unbound fact sheets produced by the Policy, Planning and Information Dissemination Unit, Ottawa, 1989.
5. Health and Welfare Canada, "Fact Sheet 1989," unbound fact sheet produced by the Policy, Planning and Information Dissemination Unit, Ottawa, 1989.
6. C. Nair, R. Karin, C. Nyers, "Healthcare and Health Status: A Canada-United States Statistical Comparison," *Health Reports 1992,* 1992, *4*(2), p. 180 (Statistics Canada Catalogue: 82-003).

Chapter Three

1. R. H. Brook and others, "Predicting The Appropriate Use of Carotid Endarterectomy, Upper Gastrointestinal Endoscopy, and Coronary Angiography," *New England Journal of Medicine,* 1990, *323*(17), pp. 1173–1177.
2. Spoken at Looking North for Health, a Families USA Foundation Forum for the Press, Washington, D.C., Oct. 30, 1989.
3. Spoken at Looking North for Health, Oct. 30, 1989.

Chapter Four

1. Data from Table 123 in Decima Research, *Decima Quarterly Report,* Fall 1987, p. 130.

2. Harris poll cited in R. J. Blendon and H. Taylor, "Views on Health Care: Public Opinion in Three Nations," *Health Affairs,* 1989, *8*(1), p. 151.

3. Data from Table 124 in Decima Research, *Decima Quarterly Report,* Fall 1987, p. 130.

4. Data from Table 125 in Decima Research, *Decima Quarterly Report,* Fall 1987, p. 130.

5. Cambridge Reports/Research International, *Health Care Trade-offs: Americans' Views on Cost, Access, and Quality* (Cambridge, Mass.: Cambridge Reports/Research International, 1990), p. 7.

6. Data from Table 157 in Decima Research, *Decima Quarterly Report,* Spring 1988, p. 166.

7. Data from Table 172 in Decima Research, *Decima Quarterly Report,* Spring 1988, p. 173.

8. Decima Research, unpublished data, Toronto.

9. Cambridge Reports/Research International, *Keeping America Healthy: Public Access to Health Care, Personal Attention to Diet* (Cambridge, Mass.: Cambridge Reports/Research International, 1992), p. 9.

Chapter Five

1. A. E. Blakeney, "Press Coverage and the Medicare Dispute," *Queen's Quarterly,* 1963, *70,* pp. 352–361.

Chapter Six

1. The material in this chapter is based on policies and programs in place in October 1989. All the provincial programs have evolved in various ways, and some details may now differ from those presented here. General program goals and activities remain the same.

2. R. A. Kane and R. L. Kane, *A Will and a Way: What the United States Can Learn from Canada About Caring for the Elderly* (New York: Columbia University Press, 1985), pp. 65–104.

3. According to a paper delivered by M. Hollander at a meeting of the Canadian Home Care Association in conjunction with the 1988 annual meeting of the Canadian Association of Gerontology.
4. R. A. Kane and R. L. Kane, "Lessons from In-Home and Community Based Care in Canada," in D. Rowland and B. Lyons (eds.), *Financing Home Care: Improving Protections for Disabled Elderly People* (Baltimore, Md.: Johns Hopkins University Press, 1991).

Chapter Seven

1. Government of British Columbia, Ministry of Health, *Ministry of Health Annual Report* (Victoria: Government of British Columbia, Ministry of Health, 1989–1990), p. 105.
2. Government of British Columbia, Ministry of Finance and Corporate Relations, *Ministry of Finance and Corporate Relations Estimates, 1989–1990* (Victoria: Government of British Columbia, Ministry of Finance and Corporate Relations, 1989–1990), pp. 116–118.
3. Government of British Columbia, Ministry of Finance and Corporate Relations, *Ministry of Finance and Corporate Relations Estimates,* 1989–1990.

Chapter Eight

1. P. Pallan, speaking at the Families USA Foundation forum, Looking North for Health, Washington, D.C., Oct. 30, 1989.
2. R. A. Kane, speaking at the same Families USA Foundation forum, Oct. 30, 1989.
3. Department of Employment and Immigration, Canada, "Immigration File," machine-readable data file (Hull: Department of Employment and Immigration, 1991).
4. M. Stevenson, E. Vayda, and P. Williams, *1986 National*

Survey of Canadian Physicians: Report to Respondents (Toronto: York University, 1987), pp. 1–7.

5. U.S. General Accounting Office, *Canadian Health Insurance: Lessons for the United States,* report to the Chairman, Committee on Government Operations, House of Representatives (Washington, D.C.: U.S. Government Printing Office, June 1991), Report No. GAO/HRD-91-90, p. 5.

6. Health and Welfare Canada, *National Expenditures 1990* (Ottawa: Policy, Planning and Information Dissemination Unit, 1990); *National Expenditures Estimates 1991* (Ottawa: Policy, Planning and Information Dissemination Unit, 1991).

7. G. J. Schieber and J. P. Poullier, "International Health Care Expenditure Trends: 1987," *Health Affairs,* 1989, *8*(3), pp. 170–177.

8. Health and Welfare Canada, *National Health Expenditures 1970–1982* (Ottawa: Policy, Planning and Information Dissemination Unit, 1984); also *National Health Expenditures 1960–1973* (published 1975); *National Health Expenditures 1960–1971* (1973); *National Health Expenditures 1975–1985* (1987); *National Health Expenditures 1975–1987* (1990); *National Health Expenditures 1990* (1990); and *National Expenditures Estimates 1991* (1991).

9. National Council of Welfare, "Health, Healthcare, and Medicare," unpublished report, National Council of Welfare, Ottawa, June 1990, p. 58.

10. R. Wilkins and O. B. Adams, "Health Expectancy in Canada, Late 1970s," in C. D'Arcy, G. Torrence, and P. New (eds.), *Health in Canadian Society: Sociological Perspectives* (2nd ed.) (Toronto: Sitzhenry and Whiteside, 1987), pp. 36–56.

11. E. J. Gallant, "Report of the Nova Scotia Royal Commission on Health Care—Towards a New Strategy," The Nova Scotia Royal Commission on Health Care, 1989, p. 20.

12. Statement of George J. Schieber, director of the Office

of Research, Health Care Financing Administration, before the Joint Economic Subcommittee on Education and
Health, May 3, 1988. From an unpublished background
paper, p. 13.

13. Statistics Canada, *Vital Statistics: Volume III, Deaths* (Ottawa: Supply and Services Canada, 1977), Catalogue 84-
206; Statistics Canada, *Life Tables, Canada and Provinces
1980–82* (Ottawa: Supply and Services Canada, 1984),
Catalogue 84:532; Canadian Centre for Health Information, Statistics Canada, unpublished 1985–1987 data.

14. D. Feeny and G. Stoddart, "Policy Options for Health
Care Technology," in D. Feeny, G. Guyatt, and P. Tugwell, *Health Care Technology: Effectiveness, Efficiency and Public Policy* (Quebec Institute for Research on Public Policy,
1986), pp. 225–226.

15. P. Manga, "Cost-Containing Medical Technology," *Health
Management Forum*, 1989, *2*(1), pp. 26–31.

16. Ontario Medical Association, *Guidelines for the Use of Coronary Thrombolysis*, 1-page fact sheet (Ottawa: Ontario Medical Association, 1988).

17. D. A. Rublee, "Medical Technology in Germany, Canada,
and the United States," *Health Affairs*, 1989, *8*(3), p. 180.

18. H. Scully, "Care for Target Groups: Can the System Ac-
commodate Special Cases?" paper presented at Health
Care in Canada: Cost Control and Rationing of Care, a
Financial Post Conference, Toronto, 1989, p. 122.

19. D. Naylor and P. Armstrong, "Guidelines for the Use of
Intravenous Thrombolytic Agents in Acute Myocardial
Infarction," *Canadian Medical Association Journal*, 1989,
140(11), p. 1289.

Chapter Nine

1. J. T. Liu, C. Regan, T. Orloff, and L. Rivera, *The Health
of America's Children 1992: Maternal and Child Health Data
Book* (Washington, D.C.: Children's Defense Fund, 1992),
p. 14.

2. National Health Care Campaign, "Selected Comparisons Between the Canadian Health Care System and the United States Health Care System: Health Care Costs, Quality, and Availability to the Average Person," charts with health statistics, Oct. 1989, p. 5.

3. Organization for Economic Development, "Health Data File," machine-readable data file (Paris: Organization for Economic Development, 1990).

4. A. Sardell, "Child Health Policy in the U.S.: The Paradox of Consensus," *Journal of Health Politics, Policy and Law,* 1990, *15*(2), p. 272.

5. A. Sardell, "Child Health Policy in the U.S.: The Paradox of Consensus," p. 272.

6. C. Nair, R. Karin, and C. Nyers, "Health Care and Health Status: A Canada–United States Statistical Comparison," *Health Reports,* 1992, *4*(2), p. 180. (Statistics Canada Catalogue: 82-003).

7. A. I. Mushlin, "Oversupply of Screening Mammography Units: Why Should Internists Care?" *Annals of Internal Medicine,* 1990, *113*(7), pp. 489–490.

8. Cited in Mushlin, "Oversupply of Screening Mammography Units."

9. R. McLelland, "Supply and Quality of Screening Mammography: A Radiologist's View," *Annals of Internal Medicine,* 1990, *113*(7), pp. 490–491.

10. Mushlin, p. 490.

11. American College of Surgeons, "Guidelines for Minimum Standards in Cardiac Surgery," *Bulletin of the American College of Surgeons,* 1991, *76*(8), p. 28.

12. H. S. Luft, J. P. Bunker, and A. C. Enthoven, "Should Operations Be Regionalized? The Empirical Relation Between Surgical Volume and Mortality," *New England Journal of Medicine,* 1979, *301*(25), p. 1364.

13. B. Patten, "Open Market, Open Heart," *Phoenix Gazette,* August 26, 1987, p. A-9.

14. Patten, "Open Market, Open Heart," p. A-10.

15. Patten, p. A-11.

16. Patten, p. A-12.

17. M. Terris quotes the Harris poll in his article "Lessons from Canada's Health Program," *Technology Review,* 1990, *93*(2), p. 29.

18. U.S. General Accounting Office, *Canadian Health Insurance: Lessons for the United States,* report to the Chairman, Committee on Government Operations, House of Representatives (Washington, D.C.: U.S. Government Printing Office, June 1991), Report No. GAO/HRD-91-90, p. 5.

19. U.S. Bureau of the Census, "A Look at Insurance Coverage," *Census and You,* 1992, *27*(9), p. 8.

20. R. G. Evans and others, "Controlling Health Expenditures — The Canadian Reality," *New England Journal of Medicine,* 1989, *320*(9), p. 572.

21. R. G. Evans, and others, "Controlling Health Expenditures — The Canadian Reality," p. 573.

22. E. Ryten, "Trends in the Demand for Medical Education in Canada," unpublished paper (Ottawa: Association of Canadian Medical Colleges, 1989).

23. U.S. Bipartisan Commission on Comprehensive Health Care, The Pepper Commission, *A Call for Action* (Washington, D.C.: U.S. Government Printing Office, 1990), p. 92.

24. Long Term Care Campaign, "The Political Impact of Long Term Care," survey conducted in 1988 by Louis Harris & Associates for Long Term Care Campaign, Washington, D.C., 1988, p. 4.

25. J. P. Firman and S. Polniaszek, "The Unaffordability of Nursing Home Insurance," a study for Families USA Foundation, January 1990, p. 5.

26. S. T. Sonnefeld, D. R. Waldo, D. R. McKusick, and J. A. Lemieux, "Projection of National Health Expenditures Through the Year 2,000," *Health Care Financing Review,* 1991, *13*(1), p. 22.

27. R. Stone, G. Cafferata, and J. Sangl, "Caregivers of the Frail Elderly: A National Profile," *The Gerontologist,* 1987, *27*(5), pp. 616–626.

28. "The Political Impact of Long Term Care," Long Term Care '88, 1987, p. 8.

29. American Medical Association, *Public Opinion on Health Care Issues 1992* (Chicago: American Medical Association, 1992), p. 13.

30. Long Term Care Campaign, "A Survey of New Hampshire Voters on Health Care and Long Term Care," conducted by Lauer, Lalley & Associates for Long Term Care Campaign, Washington, D.C., November 1991.

31. Long Term Care Campaign, "The Political Impact of Long Term Care," survey conducted by R. L. Associates for Long Term Care Campaign, Washington, D.C., 1988, p. 5.

Index

187